Podiatry

D0864178

Dedication

This book is dedicated to the memory of the real-life patients who are named in this book as *Matthew Johnson* in Chapter 12 and as *Margaret Knowles* in Chapter 18.

Podiatry: Case-based psychology

Anne Mandy
Kevin Lucas
Jodie Lucas

With Janet McInnes
Chair
Society of Chiropodists and Podiatrists
UK

WILEY-BLACKWELL

This edition first published 2009
© 2009, John Wiley & Sons Ltd.

Wiley-Blackwell is an imprint of John Wiley & Sons, formed by the merger of Wiley's global
Scientific, Technical and Medical business with Blackwell Publishing.

Registered office
John Wiley & Sons Ltd, The Atrium, Southern Gate, Chichester, West Sussex, PO19 8SQ,
United Kingdom

Editorial office
John Wiley & Sons Ltd, The Atrium, Southern Gate, Chichester, West Sussex, PO19 8SQ,
United Kingdom

For details of our global editorial offices, for customer services and for information about how to
apply for permission to reuse the copyright material in this book please see our website at
www.wiley.com/wiley-blackwell.

The right of the author to be identified as the author of this work has been asserted in accordance
with the Copyright, Designs and Patents Act 1988.

All rights reserved. No part of this publication may be reproduced, stored in a retrieval system, or
transmitted, in any form or by any means, electronic, mechanical, photocopying, recording or
otherwise, except as permitted by the UK Copyright, Designs and Patents Act 1988, without the
prior permission of the publisher.

Wiley also publishes its books in a variety of electronic formats. Some content that appears in
print may not be available in electronic books.

Designations used by companies to distinguish their products are often claimed as trademarks. All
brand names and product names used in this book are trade names, service marks, trademarks or
registered trademarks of their respective owners. The publisher is not associated with any product
or vendor mentioned in this book. This publication is designed to provide accurate and
authoritative information in regard to the subject matter covered. It is sold on the understanding
that the publisher is not engaged in rendering professional services. If professional advice or other
expert assistance is required, the services of a competent professional should be sought.

Library of Congress Cataloging-in-Publication Data:

Mandy, Anne.
  Podiatry : case-based psychology / Anne Mandy, Kevin Lucas, Jodie Lucas ; with
Janet McInnes.
    p. ; cm.
  Includes bibliographical references and index.
  ISBN 978-0-470-51963-9 (pbk. : alk. paper) 1. Podiatry – Psychological aspects.
2. Podiatry – Social aspects. 3. Foot – Diseases – Psychological aspects. I. Lucas, Kevin, 1954-
II. Lucas, Jodie. III. Title.
  [DNLM: 1. Foot Diseases – psychology. 2. Case Reports. 3. Foot Diseases – therapy.
4. Physician-Patient Relations. 5. Podiatry – methods. 6. Socioeconomic Factors. WE 880
M273p 2009]
  RD563.M356 2009
  617.5′85 – dc22

                                                                              2009004166

A catalogue record for this book is available from the British Library.

Typeset in 10.5/12.5 Minion by Laserwords Private Limited, Chennai, India.
Printed and bound in Singapore by Fabulous Printers Pte Ltd.

1 2009

Contents

About the authors

Anne Mandy PhD, MSc, BSc(Hons), DPodM, Cert Ed
Reader
Clinical Research Centre
School of Health Professions
University of Brighton

Kevin Lucas DPhil, BA, PGDipHEd, PGCAP, HMFPHMed, RMN, RGN
Senior Lecturer in Psychology Applied to Healthcare
School of Health Professions
University of Brighton

Jodie Lucas BSc(Hons), MChS
Podiatrist
Seaview Project
Southwater Centre
Hastings

Janet McInnes BSc(Hons), DPodM, Cert Ed
Head of Podiatry
School of Health Professions
University of Brighton
and
Chair, Society of Chiropodists and Podiatrists UK

Preface

If one does not understand a person, one tends to regard him as a fool.

Carl Jung

The aim of this book is to provide a problem- and case-based approach to understanding psychological and social difficulties that people often experience and present to practitioners. To our knowledge, this is the first book of its kind for undergraduate podiatry students.

In everyday clinical practice, podiatrists will encounter patients who have a range of problems that need to be understood. In the United Kingdom, the current undergraduate curricula for both podiatry and physiotherapy do contain modules on health psychology. However, the great majority of these densely packed courses are concerned with topics such as anatomy, physiology, pathology and pharmacology. Whilst a good working knowledge of these subjects is clearly essential for safe and effective clinical practice, we would argue that insufficient consideration of patients' psychological and emotional needs is given in the overall training of allied health professionals. It is our experience that once in clinical practice students are often struck by the complexity of needs exhibited by real people as opposed to hypothetical patients employed to illustrate disease processes, and certainly by the multifactorial nature of real-life cases compared to the models provided in undergraduate training (that is each other). No single volume can properly prepare student practitioners for the range of issues that they will encounter, even in the early years of their practice, but we have attempted to provide real-life examples which cover some common situations that students will meet.

Although based in podiatric practice, this book is not intended only to be a podiatry textbook. The scenarios and patients it describes could readily be transferred to the work of physiotherapists, nurses and other health care professionals.

The clinical case studies and vignettes presented have been designed to meet a variety of needs, including those of students and clinicians. They will realistically assist in preparing podiatry students and podiatrists intellectually and emotionally for situations encountered in practice. The book as a whole represents an attempt to empower clinicians to develop their clinical skills.

How to use this book

The cases presented are based on real patients that we have treated over several decades of clinical practice. Anonymised, they provide a vehicle for learning and illustrate the importance of understanding psychosocial issues in the context of holistic podiatric care. By contrast, the two podiatrists introduced in this book are entirely fictitious but possess characteristics which merit consideration.

It is not necessary to read this book in the order in which it is written. Students are encouraged to read chapters which are relevant to their learning and clinical experience, as each of the scenarios is self-contained yet makes reference to other sections of the book as and when necessary.

Each chapter contains challenges for a student to consider. An outline of important issues is provided, but these are not intended to be exhaustive and the student is encouraged to think around the problems and possible outcomes.

This approach has determined the format in which the book is written: the main chapters are organised as individual patient case studies with the relevant psychological theory attached. Attention is also given to socio-psychological issues pertinent to both newly qualified and experienced podiatric practitioners. Theory is thus explained in the context of the presenting patient in a spirit of problem-based learning, enabling the reader to acquire knowledge and skills that would otherwise be gained more slowly. This book is designed to be an introduction to important applied psychology in clinical practice. Where a more extensive understanding of psychological theory is required, the reader is referred to appropriate sources. This volume is designed for self-directed learning but may also be used as a basis for Action Learning Sets or informal discussion groups, where cases will stimulate interest, dialogue and debate. Each section poses questions for the student to consider and provides an explanation of key issues. The learning activities and challenges will draw on theoretical models underpinning psychological theory. These are then applied to podiatry in a clinically useful way.

Acknowledgements

We would like to thank Dr Philip Mandy for the original work that he contributed to Chapter 1 and Dr Simon Otter for the original work in Chapter 24.

Introduction: Using case-based learning

Case-based learning is an educational strategy (Colliver, 2000) in which the learner works in a self-directed manner towards the understanding or resolution of a practice-related issue. The learning process encourages reflective, critical and active learning and enhances the acquisition of clinical reasoning, critical thinking and judgement. Active learning empowers and inspires the learner by providing opportunities for success, achievement and the enjoyment of learning.

The practice of podiatry is as much an art as a science. Each patient presents as a unique individual and multidimensional challenge which requires the podiatrist to have a cognitive model for clinical reasoning and professional skills (Cote, 1993). Through the exploration of issues presented by the patients, the learner engages in the process of critical thinking while applying and integrating new information, and uses clinical reasoning to determine the best outcome for the patient. It is our intention that podiatry students using this book will embark on an education using a strategy that will not only result in a professional qualification but also help them to begin to develop a basis for lifelong learning, which should result in greater clinical success and satisfaction.

The role of the student

All students need to develop the professional skills and work habits of an autonomous professional clinician. This development results from the experience gained by working with patients. The process of acquiring the appropriate information and skills needed to undertake clinical reasoning and decision-making is multifactorial and complex, and for some students this transition is difficult to address. Students and therapists need to be able to apply appropriate theory in the context of complex situations with the added constraints of the realities of clinical practice. The patient scenarios contained within this text require the student to consider the issues presented by the characters in order to have an improved understanding of the patient's needs.

Each section begins with a summary of information describing the content of the case. A clinical podiatric presentation for each character is then provided for the student to consider.

The characters in this book are based on patients and colleagues drawn from the authors' own professional practice. Changes have been made in order to protect their identities.

Health psychology and the podiatry student

Up until the end of the last century, much of the curriculum for podiatry students was concerned with the scientific and theoretical basis for clinical work. Theories underpinning patient behaviour were largely ignored in the belief that exposure to clinical experience would suffice. This *medical model* has had an enormous influence over podiatric education and practice. The model demands a mechanistic approach, which regards the symptoms of illness as the failure of an anatomical structure or of a system. Health and disease are considered to be contrasting states and are thus defined solely in mechanistic terms. In these terms, *health* is exemplified by the body being in good working order, while any deviation from the norm is seen as *disease*. In the view of the medical model, treatment is provided to restore physiological function or to remove faulty structures.

In the 1970s, Engel (1977) proposed a bio-psychosocial model of health, suggesting that, while pathogens may be responsible for changing health status, behavioural, psychological and social factors also represent equally powerful influences on a person's state of health or illness. In addition, recovery from illness is now known to be strongly mediated by psychosocial factors, such as personality, coping styles and psychological well-being. It is also now well established that an individual's environment and social networks fundamentally influence their health status, prognosis in the case of disease and life expectancy.

Students in podiatry need to learn to appreciate the complexity of patients' needs that are beyond the simple pathology that instigates their arrival at the clinic.

Whilst we all have a general understanding of the terms *illness* and *disease*, it is important to have a common understanding of these terms for the purposes of this book. Our definition of *illness* is rooted as much in the individual's experience of being unwell as in the pathological state of an organ or system. Moreover, it is important to recognise that it is common for a patient to have a disease without experiencing illness, for example in pre-clinical cancers. Conversely, it is possible for a patient to experience illness in the absence of organic pathology, for example in anxiety states or depression.

In recent years, health psychology addressed many aspects of the experience of illness and distress, such as pain, addiction and bereavement. Some podiatry students may encounter these experiences in their own lives, but not all podiatry students will have done so at the time of their professional training. It is therefore important that podiatry students appreciate the magnitude of the impact such factors have on their patients, and it is this appreciation that this book aims to engender

The relationship between any practitioner and patient depends on many factors, including gender, age, culture, social class and the nature of the therapeutic interaction. The nature of the therapeutic interaction in turn varies according to the professional discipline. The relationship between a podiatrist and their patients is in some ways rather different from that associated with other disciplines. First, the time that podiatrists spend with their patients on a one-to-one basis is frequently longer than that of other professionals. This often results in patients using the podiatrist as a confidant.

Second, in podiatric practice, patients rarely present with serious or life-threatening illnesses. Podiatric patients usually have considerable understanding of their conditions and may well have experienced those conditions for a protracted period. The quality of the professional–patient relationship is thus much more equal than in many other settings.

It maybe useful at this point to consider notions of health education and health promotion in relation to podiatric practice. Much of the current interaction between podiatrists and their patients may be seen in terms of health education, that is the dissemination of information pertinent to both the patient's individual condition and their health status in general. On the other hand, health promotion is concerned with a wider view of an individual's health. Thus, it may be necessary for a clinician to accept that a patient's priorities may differ from that of their own or, indeed, what may be 'best' for the patient's podiatric condition. Such a holistic approach is a key feature of health-promotion activity and has been explored extensively elsewhere (Lucas and Lloyd, 2005). The implications for podiatric practice are discussed in terms of compliance and concordance in Chapter 5.

However, the clinical environment in which podiatrists practise is not always conducive to accommodating some of the patient's psychological needs. The clinical layout of the practice and the use of surgical instruments, and podiatric treatments, are reminiscent of those of dentists, and certainly do not create an ideal environment in which to develop a therapeutic relationship. The clinical environment and nature of podiatric practice may particularly affect new patients. New patients are exposed to a range of unusual sights, noises, smells and procedures, which may make them feel anxious. The podiatrist should always endeavour to put patients at their ease, explain carefully what they should expect from the consultation and use minimal intervention where possible. When designing clinical environments, efforts to 'humanise' what may appear to be a cold and sterile surgery are likely to be much appreciated by podiatric patients. Similarly, the podiatrist should be aware that the conventional position adopted for treatment (where the podiatrist is seated at the feet of the patient) is not ideal for interviewing and history-taking, when maintaining eye contact is of considerable importance. However, most patients become familiar and comfortable with the environment after the initial visit.

Podiatrists work in a range of environments, including the NHS, private practice, through commercial high-street companies, in occupational health departments and in education and research. While such variety offers many opportunities to achieve job satisfaction, some research suggests that the need for collegiality and identified roles within teams is key to its realisation (Mandy, A., 2000). These issues are explored further in Chapter 6.

The characters presented within this book are based on real people. While it is unlikely that any one podiatrist's caseload would contain patients with such a complex range of problems at any one time, the characters are used as a vehicle to illustrate a range of issues which most podiatrists will encounter in the course of their professional lives. It is not the aim of this book to make all podiatrists into quasi-psychologists. Its aim is to introduce the student to some important psychological concepts that may influence and improve their clinical practice and provide the clinician-in-training with skills that will enhance clinical reasoning by better understanding their patients' needs.

Chapter 1

The sociology of podiatry as a profession

Amateurs built the Ark, but professionals built the Titanic.

Anon

The aim of this chapter is to provide a brief sociological perspective of podiatry, and of its associated implications for podiatric practice.

Similarities between podiatry and medicine

An intra-professional hierarchy has long been recognised within medicine. Merton *et al.* (1956), Becker *et al.* (1961) and Schartzbaum *et al.* (1973) all describe such a hierarchy, which is led by specialist surgery, followed by general surgery and thereafter various divisions of internal medicine. General practice and dermatology follow, with psychiatry generally being regarded as the least prestigious branch of the profession (Abbott, 1981). Within the health care professions, a hierarchy has begun to develop which closely mirrors that found in medicine. For example, podiatric surgery has an extensive history but has only recently developed into a speciality in its own right. Borthwick (2000) describes the issue of podiatric surgery and the boundaries of clinical practice. The training to become a podiatric surgeon requires postgraduate study and clinical practice in order to meet the requirements of the Faculty of Podiatric Surgery. Similarly, there are emergent specialisms in podiatric medicine, including rheumatology, diabetic care, paediatrics and biomechanics. Observation suggests that those podiatrists who specialise are deemed to be higher in the professional hierarchy than are those who remain generalists. It may be salutary to note that, by contrast, there is as yet no 'speciality' for the podiatric care of older patients, despite the fact that older people represent the majority of our patients.

Podiatry and other health professions

In general, podiatry as a profession has had a long and convoluted history. It was solely in search of recognition (and hence status) that a few of the many bodies formerly representing podiatrists came together under the Board of Registration of Medical Auxiliaries' (BRMA) recognition in 1942. It was not until 18 years later that a 1960 Act of Parliament established the Council for Professions Supplementary to Medicine (CPSM) as the statutory and regulatory body for these professions. Each professional discipline within the Council was then given its own regulatory board.

The Health Professions Council (HPC) replaced the CPSM in April 2002, and there are no longer separate boards for each profession. Within the HPC, interdisciplinary hierarchies are still seen to exist. Yet as the professions concerned are roughly comparable in terms of income, power and education, such hierarchies cannot be explained by traditional criteria.

Early sociologists employed a number of approaches in attempts to explain the process of professionalisation; these theoretical orientations are outside the focus of this book, but are described in considerable detail elsewhere (Carr-Saunders and Wilson, 1933; Parsons, 1939). Later, Greenwood (1957) considered the successive steps any occupation goes through in order to achieve professional status. He suggests that the process involves:

1. Doing (full-time) something that needs to be done. The sick were always nursed, but technical and organisational developments created nursing as a profession.
2. Early practitioners (or the public) campaign for the establishment of a formal training school. While not all schools originated in universities (e.g. in the case of public-sector administrators, city planners and accountants), they all eventually sought support from universities.
3. Proponents of prescribed training, and the first alumni, combine to form a professional association.
4. Pressure is exerted in order to win legal protection of the job territory and its sustaining code of ethics.

Eventually, rules are made to eliminate the unqualified, to reduce internal competition and to protect clients. The ideal of service then becomes embodied in a formal code of ethics (Wilensky, 1964). Later, Storch and Stinson (1988) suggested that the two main distinguishing characteristics of a profession are a body of abstract knowledge and an ideal of service.

Professionalism and professional status

While status differences create gross hierarchical structures, they do not automatically produce the exact *order* of hierarchy, which is generated by measures of honour, power, wealth and knowledge. Abbott (1981) maintains that income, power and client status are important factors in determining such order. Yet income may be an unreliable determinant of status; for example, within NHS medicine, salaries are similar irrespective of the area of specialism, yet different specialisms clearly have different status.

However, Abbott also suggests complexity as an alternative basis for determining intra-professional status; put simply, high status is attributed to non-routine work. General practitioners refer difficult, non-routine cases to specialists, who handle them or in turn pass them on to even more specialist practitioners. Conversely, routine aspects of professional practice are often delegated to the paraprofessional level (Freidson, 1970). In the case of podiatry, patients may be referred 'upwards' to specialist podiatric surgeons or 'downwards' to foot care assistants.

Most foot conditions worsen with age, and systemic complications are more likely in older people. It is therefore the case that the majority of patients in receipt of podiatry care are over 50 years of age. Many authors have noted the ageism intrinsic to Western society. Given the current status of podiatry in relation to other health professions, Abbott (1981) may be correct in citing client status as an indicator of professional status. If this is the case, then podiatric practitioners must develop not only their own professional status but also coping mechanisms for dealing with the attitudes of other professionals in the meantime.

Education and knowledge have always been emphasised by professions seeking higher status (Larson, 1977). Abbott (1981) maintains that 'the overall correlation of education and social status is undeniable'. However, this fails to explain the relative status of professional groups whose education and levels of knowledge may be similar, for example podiatrists and physiotherapists. Even though both receive education of a similar level (in some institutions physiotherapy and podiatry students share classes), the British public perceives physiotherapists as being of a higher status than podiatrists (Mandy, P., 2000).

Two other factors may also influence the status of a professional group: the gender balance of the profession and the nature of the professional practice. Professions having a higher proportion of female members consistently have lower status than professions that are male-dominated. A frequently cited example is the relationship of nursing to medicine. However, medical school intakes in the United Kingdom have been balanced by gender for many years, and certain areas of nursing (notably psychiatry) have always attracted roughly equal numbers of men and women. Nevertheless, in both professions women are under-represented in senior positions. Thus, Abbott's fourth factor, the nature of professional activity, may provide better explanations of the hierarchical structure of the health professions. However, it is this factor that is by far the least investigated.

Professional autonomy

For a paramedical profession to attain autonomy, it must concern itself with a discrete area of work that can be separated from the main body of medicine. It must also be able to practise that area of work without routine contact with, or dependence on, doctors. From an early period, podiatry has provided services through an occupational structure separate from medicine. This is also true of opticians, speech therapists and speech pathologists. But despite gaining relative autonomy of practice, higher status has not yet followed.

Monopolisation is an established tactic for restricting the number of competitors and ensuring the maintenance of a profession. Dentists gained a similar monopoly with professional closure in 1921, despite continued conflict with medicine. At the time of writing, podiatry has still to acquire any such legal privileges. A profession maintains its position by recognising that changes in medical knowledge and technology, as well as changing patterns of morbidity and mortality, result in important modifications (Elton, 1977). Some roles become obsolete, others emerge: specialisation breeds occupational homogeneity, and groups with conflicting interest appear, thus weakening professional solidarity and potentially threatening a profession's dominant position. External challenges come from different sources: other occupations, whether they are in direct competition or in a position of subordination to the dominant group, also try to improve their status and increase their work autonomy.

Historically, dominant professions such as medicine and law have experienced inter- and intra-professional conflicts as well as conflict with the state. Their responses have involved both their clientele and the recruitment of 'suitable' new members in the maintenance of occupational cohesiveness, a process known as 'patrolling the entrance gate'. In organising formal training and in instituting qualifying procedures, occupations seeking professional status assert that only their members have the competence to perform certain tasks or to deliver certain services. Finally, professional groups engage in political activity to gain state recognition and to develop a legal monopoly of certain activities.

Practitioner–patient relationships

In considering the nature of practice, it is important to consider the relationship between the professional and the patient. Parsons (1951) portrays the doctor–patient relationship as one of reciprocity, in which the doctor and patient have certain obligations and privileges attached to their respective roles. Morgan *et al.* (1991) suggest that Parsons' analysis of the relationship is based on the two parties being socialised in their roles. The patient, as part of the obligations attached to the sick role, is expected to seek technically competent help usually from a doctor and to trust the doctor and to accept that the doctor is a competent help giver. Conversely, the doctor is expected:

■ to act in accordance with the health needs of his or her patient
■ to follow the rules of professional conduct
■ to use a high degree of expertise and knowledge
■ to remain objective and emotionally neutral.

This reciprocity is particularly pertinent in the case of Charles Walters, a patient described in Chapter 7.

A more detailed analysis of the doctor–patient relationship was developed by Szasz and Hollender (1956), and is considered in greater detail in Chapter 4.

The practitioner–patient relationship will be explored later in the book in the context of the character of Suzi Dalton in Chapter 5.

Podiatry patients are often prepared to assume an active role in their treatment. Friedson (1971) presents patients as active and critical in rejecting professional services, when they contradicted their own conceptions of illness. In some cases, he argues, patients perceived their own and other lay alternatives to be superior to professional medical opinion.

When examining podiatric care, it is interesting to consider these issues. Patients are able to observe the whole treatment process to their feet and, indeed, often attempt their own treatment, sometimes with painful or damaging results. They have a clear idea of both what they think they require and how it should be achieved. By their ability to observe the podiatrist at work, they can take an active role in their own treatment. Thus, Friedson's analysis may be applied accurately to podiatry. Clinicians are advised to consider carefully the patient's social and cultural context. The character of Sheetal Joshi (Chapter 9) considers this issue in greater detail.

People are able to examine their own feet. As a result, patients attending podiatric services will have formed a view of the aetiology of their conditions and will attend for treatment rather than preventative monitoring. Monitoring is an important part of podiatric care, particularly for patients suffering from diabetes. Such patients often experience complications, such as peripheral arterial disease and its associated neuropathy. Minor cuts or abrasions, if untreated, may result in ulceration and ultimately amputation of the toes or limb. In addition regular monitoring of the vascular status of the patient may identify such complications early enough to initiate treatment which will minimise their effects. These issues will be discussed further in the characters of George Archer in Chapter 21 and Charles Walters in Chapter 7.

Such monitoring requires well-developed communication skills on the part of the podiatrist. Communication skills and communication theory are discussed in the context of the characters Suzi Dalton in Chapter 5, Enid Hilton in Chapter 10 and James Watt in Chapter 8.

Professionalisation is pertinent to podiatric practice, where the desire to improve professional status may be in danger of overshadowing the intrinsic altruism of the occupation. Perhaps ironically, there is no evidence that an increase in professional status improves the practitioner's self-esteem or feelings of professional worth. Traditionally, high-status professionals may also suffer from low self-esteem, and the prevalence of psychological problems among 'higher' professionals has reached alarming proportions.

Nevertheless, social status has profound effects upon human relationships, and this issue is discussed in the context of the character Bill Canning in Chapter 11. Podiatry currently has comparatively low professional status, partly because it does not meet some established status criteria, but mainly because much of its work can be routine and less than glamorous. However, this should not deter its practitioners: if podiatrists take an objective view of podiatry's position and accept the reality that expert foot care is, and increasingly will be, required, then the profession could prosper. Paradoxically, by not attempting to pursue the criteria for high status but instead establishing its own professional niche and improving its own expertise, the professional standing of podiatry could rise.

Chapter 2

Issues faced by newly qualified podiatrists

Far and away the best prize that life offers is the chance to work hard at work worth doing.

Theodore Roosevelt

Jenny Fraser exemplifies some of the problems and frustrations that newly qualified podiatrists may experience. She raises issues about coping with the demands of a new job, sources of occupational stress and ways in which she can effectively deal with her new situation.

Jenny is a newly qualified podiatrist who graduated from university last summer. She is an enthusiastic and cheerful young woman who always wanted to be a podiatrist and is thrilled at the prospect of commencing her new career. She has recently taken up her first post as a junior podiatrist working for the state health provider. Jenny has returned to her parents' home after a period of three years at university. She is finding the constraints of home life difficult after her independence as a student. She is also having to build a new social life because most of her school friends chose employment in the university towns where they studied.

Factors influencing Jenny's behaviour

Jenny chose to take up employment near home principally because she has a large student loan that she has to repay. Jenny was particularly attracted to her current job because of the variety of work it offers and the range of experiences she would encounter. The job includes community, hospital, domiciliary and some administrative duties.

However, on some days of the week Jenny has to travel between clinic sites, which are some distance apart, and this often involves her missing her lunch break. Jenny is thoroughly enjoying her job but finds the amount of paperwork and administration involved in her job irritating and excessive. She was not anticipating this aspect of the work, and finds it an unexpected burden. She is uncertain why she has to complete certain tasks and what happens to the information that she collects. She finds that in trying to keep up with all the administration and paperwork she often runs late with her patients' appointments, and by the end of the day she is quite behind schedule. One of the consequences of running late is that some of the patients become irritated and demanding, which causes Jenny to become anxious and frustrated.

The environment in which Jenny now works is very different from that of the university. She no longer works alongside friends and colleagues and finds working in single-chair clinics lonely. The only contact she has with her professional colleagues is on two afternoons per month when she works in the orthotics laboratory. The reception and ancillary staff, who support her clinical work at the various sites, are all extraordinarily warm and helpful. However, Jenny misses the professional discussion, support and friendship she had whilst at university. These difficulties will inevitably be exacerbated when trying to help certain patients. This is illustrated in the cases of James Watt (Chapter 8) and Margaret Knowles (Chapter 18).

In the case of James Watt, Jenny needs to learn how to deal with patients who may be aggressive and demanding, without becoming upset. Much of the resilience necessary to achieve this may be acquired through good communication skills and skilled patient management. In the case of Margaret Knowles, it is essential for Jenny to be able to set treatment objectives which meet Margaret's needs at the time of presentation.

The podiatry department is also undergoing a period of reorganisation and staff change. There are currently two members of staff on maternity leave and one unfilled vacancy. There are efficiency savings enforced, and the podiatry budget is currently slightly overspent. Whilst not being paid as a Senior II, Jenny has been asked to take on the duties usually performed by more senior colleagues.

Challenge 1: Identify the likely sources of stress for Jenny in her new job

Workload and time pressures are strongly correlated with emotional exhaustion and burnout (Lee and Ashforth, 1996). A study of newly qualified podiatrists in the United Kingdom (Mandy, A., 2000) further supported this finding. The early post-qualification period is a challenging time when professional, time-management and general organisational skills are being developed. There are several ways in which work can be stressful. These include organisational problems, such as insufficient back-up, long or unsociable hours, poor status, low pay and limited promotion prospects, as well as uncertainty and insecurity of employment. Moreover, issues such as unclear role specifications, role conflict, unrealistically high self-expectations (perfectionism), an inability to influence decision-making, frequent clashes with superiors, isolation from colleagues and the support that they can offer, lack of variety, poor communication, inadequate leadership, conflicts with colleagues, inability to finish a job and fighting unnecessary battles may also contribute to stress at work.

Lack of control over work has been identified as a source of stress that may lead to poor health. Many studies have found that heavy job demand, and low control, or decreased decision freedom lead to job dissatisfaction, mental strain and cardiovascular disease (Sutton and Kahn, 1984; Sauter *et al.*, 1989). Work by Mandy *et al.* (2007) suggests that some podiatrists report that the routine nature of their work, their perceived low status and the lack of financial remuneration were sources of frustration. These findings echoed the results reported by Farndon *et al.* (2002), who found that the most frequently reported areas of clinical practice included simple palliative care that did not utilise the practitioner's complete range of clinical skills. Macdonald and Capewell (2001) report that NHS podiatrists express frustration when carrying out low-skill tasks.

Research has found that participating actively in the planning and execution of work tasks reduces stress and hence improves health status (Israel *et al.*, 1989). A study by Jackson (1983) found that simple attendance at staff meetings (non-active participation) did not of itself influence perceived job stress. However, those people who participated actively within staff meetings reported lower job stress, improved job satisfaction and lower absenteeism. Similarly, Israel *et al.* (1989) conclude that the ability to control or influence work factors is linked to the incidence of cardiovascular disease and to psychosomatic disorders, depression and job dissatisfaction.

Role conflict can exist in many forms. There may be conflict between the job and the employee's personal values. Roles which are not clearly defined are termed *ambiguous*, and are sources of conflict, which is associated with lower productivity, increased tension, dissatisfaction and work stress (Lindquist and Whitehead, 1986). Role ambiguity occurs when insufficient information is available to perform the job in a satisfactory manner; it therefore obstructs the development of goals that direct work behaviour.

Since the early 1990s, there has been a strong political imperative in the United Kingdom to develop professional roles, thereby blurring professional boundaries and emphasising patient/client-centred care delivery. This in turn has led to major changes in professional work patterns (Colyer, 2004) and has involved a process of reduction of professional direction and autonomy. This process is called *deprofessionalisation*. Deprofessional-isation reduces a worker's professional discretion and autonomy and thus their capacity to work in the patient's best interest. It is acknowledged that the health care professions have never been static in terms of their own disciplinary boundaries, nor in their role or status in society. Health care provision has been defined by changing societal expectations and beliefs, new ways of perceiving health and illness, the introduction of a range of technologies and by the formal recognition of particular groups through the introduction of education and regulation. It has also been shaped by both interprofessional and profession–state relationships forged over time (Nancarrow and Borthwick, 2005). However, for some practitioners such changes are unsettling and can lead to dissatisfaction, particularly when staff are new. In such cases, it is important that staff feel supported.

Every podiatry department will have a slightly different induction process and period, ranging from the very simple, brief explanation of health and safety procedures to a six-month induction. In the most supportive departments, new members of staff are gradually introduced to all aspects of the job within the institution. The advantage of continued support, supervision and mentoring of staff at all levels is now widely acknowledged.

In addition, most professional codes of practice contain an expectation that staff should practise within ethical guidelines, making it essential to be able to voice concerns about patient care and patient services. In order for this to be possible, professionals need to develop confidence and assertiveness.

Effective time management requires the ability to cope with all elements of the job within a specified time. Time management includes clarification of job responsibilities, duties and roles followed by the appropriate allocation of time to each of these components. Skills may then be developed in prioritising, planning and delegation.

Prioritising work also ensures that important issues are addressed first. Identification of *time robbers*, such as unnecessary meetings and phone calls, will reduce wasted time.

Challenge 2: What strategies can Jenny employ to ensure that she remains optimistic and healthy within her job?

Some of Jenny's friends from university work in a neighbouring health authority. At a recent reunion, they reported very different experiences from Jenny's. Most of them had experienced an extensive induction programme and had been allocated a mentor, who was an experienced practitioner. There is an organised programme of staff meetings, a programme of continuous professional development and various courses available for staff. A new scheme for clinical supervision aimed at providing mutual support is being developed by the entire staff team. The exposure of this contrasting situation offers Jenny a different and more positive perspective to employment.

Lazarus (1991) identifies at least two strategies for reducing work-related stress:

1. Alter the working conditions so that they are less stressful or more conducive to effective coping. This strategy is most appropriate for large numbers of workers working under severe conditions. Examples include altering physical annoyances such as noise levels, or changing organisational decision-making processes to include employees. In Jenny's case, it is important that she be encouraged to contribute her opinions and suggestions at staff meetings, and where possible she be involved in teamwork.
2. Help is made available to employees to enable them to acquire more effective coping strategies for situations that are impossible or difficult to change.

Conclusion

In order for Jenny to enjoy her job, she must maintain a healthy balance between her work and her social life. Many individuals find that their social life is closely associated with their professional life, and there are many special-interest groups in podiatry through which Jenny could meet colleagues with similar interests. Developing a programme of continuous professional development will contribute significantly to her job satisfaction.

Chapter 3

The effects of culture on behavioural change

We are indeed much more than what we eat, but what we eat can nevertheless help us to be much more than what we are.

Adelle Davis

Joseph Camilleri is a 53-year-old man who moved to the United Kingdom from Sliema in Malta when he was in his late forties. Joseph and his wife, Ellicia, left Sliema when their only daughter married an Englishman and set up home in south London. He specifically chose to live in this part of London because there is a discrete Maltese community which engages in the traditional *festas*. The Maltese *festa* has carved its niche in London, supported by the organisation of a cohesive Maltese community. Malta's best-loved and historically important feast is *Il-Vitorja*, the feast of Our Lady of Victories, and it occurs on the Saturday nearest 8th September. The festivities recall Malta's victories against great odds and over adversity in the sieges of 1565 and 1940–1942. Despite the passage of time, the feast still reflects the values and beliefs that the Maltese people cherish in their homeland and preserve wherever fate and fortune has taken them. Feeling part of, and being able to participate in, the familiar Maltese celebrations is very important to Joseph and his wife.

Since settling in London, Joseph has been employed as a bus driver. Obese for a number of years, he has suffered from insulin-dependent diabetes since he was 11 years of age. Although his diabetes has been moderately well controlled, he has had some podiatric complications, including a neuropathy that affects his lower limbs.

In 2007, it was estimated that there were 194 million people with diabetes in the adult population of the seven regions of the International Diabetes Federation (IDF). In 2008, this figure had risen to 246 million. In 2007, it was estimated that 7.3% of adults aged 20–79 in all IDF member countries had diabetes. The Western Pacific Region and the European Region have the highest number of people with diabetes, approximately 67 and 53 million respectively. The highest rate of diabetes prevalence is to be found in the North American region (9.2%) followed by the European Region (8.4%).

Type 2 diabetes constitutes about 85% to 95% of all diabetes cases in developed countries and accounts for an even higher percentage in developing countries. Diabetes continues to affect ever-increasing numbers of people around the world, and is acknowledged as a global epidemic. Despite this, public awareness of the disorder remains low.

Podiatric presentation

Joseph had recently noticed an unpleasant odour when he removed his shoes, and had found a redness surrounding an area of hard skin. He had tried to treat himself using bathroom surgery by picking at the callus with a pair of scissors, which exposed a small hole, 2 cm in diameter. This alarmed him and he contacted his local podiatry clinic, which gave him an emergency appointment. The podiatrist confirmed the development of an ulcer under the fifth metatarsal head on his right foot.

Factors influencing Joseph's behaviour

Malta is a small island in the Mediterranean which has one of the highest levels of diabetes in Europe (Rocchiccioli *et al.*, 2005). It is reported that 10% of the Maltese population has diabetes compared with only 2–3% on the nearby mainland of Europe (Rocchiccioli *et al.*, 2005). Nevertheless, the treatment of diabetes is less developed than is the case in Western Europe (Formosa, 2008), and amputation is far more common. Foot ulceration is the most common cause of non-traumatic amputation of the lower limb (Rocchiccioli *et al.*, 2005).

Genetic factors are partly responsible for the higher prevalence of diabetes in Malta. Because of its strategic importance, the island has experienced many hostile invasions in the past. The history of repeated sieges has resulted in periods of food shortages followed by periods of relative plenty. People who were genetically more able to cope in times of famine thus had an advantage over those who were not. This has become known as Thrifty Genotype Theory, which suggests that Maltese people are particularly vulnerable to diabetes during times in which food is plentiful (Savona-Ventura, 2005). As marriage outside the island is uncommon, this genotype has proliferated.

In addition, the traditional Maltese diet is different from that typical of other Mediterranean countries, largely as a result of the mixed cultural heritage associated with repeated occupation by other nations. Most recently the strong British presence on the island since World War II has introduced a preference for high-fat, low-fibre and refined sugars, most recently augmented by fast-food outlets. The strongly Roman Catholic faith of the Maltese people is reflected in the large number of *festas*, or religious celebrations, which are marked by eating, drinking and general festivity. These events are enormously important in the culture of the Maltese, and the tradition has helped to maintain intergenerational solidarity. It is known that the Maltese maintain these traditions for several generations following emigration to other parts of the world.

Influenced by his many acquaintances back home, Joseph believes that amputation is an inevitable consequence of his lower limb's condition.

Challenge 1: How will Joseph's religious and cultural background influence the advice you offer regarding his diet and lifestyle?

It is important to understand the importance of religious and cultural influences. Although Joseph is no longer living in Malta, he socialises with the Maltese community in London and participates in traditional Maltese celebrations and festivities. The so-called Mediterranean diet is a modern nutritional model originally inspired by the traditional eating patterns of some of the countries of the Mediterranean Basin, particularly Greece and southern Italy. The diet is often cited as beneficial because it is low in saturated fat, high in monounsaturated fat and high in fibre. The Mediterranean diet is one that is generally recommended to people with diabetes; Joseph should be encouraged to follow this type of diet.

Common to the traditional diets of those specific regions are a high consumption of fruit and vegetables, bread, wheat and other cereals, olive oil, fish and red wine. However, at times when there are celebrations, Joseph will feel the need to participate and relax his dietary regime. It would be unreasonable to expect Joseph not to participate, as this is an important part of his life. Therefore, there needs to be negotiated agreement and a realistic approach to such events. It would be advantageous for Joseph to liaise with the dietitian and diabetes nurse before the *festas* in order that he may participate in the celebrations without detriment to his health.

Challenge 2: What professional dilemma does this present to the podiatrist?

The distinction between compliance, adherence and concordance is described in Chapter 7. This scenario also raises issues which are relevant to the nature of health promotion. Were Joseph to be empowered to make an informed choice about his diabetes, it would be entirely possible that he might decide that his cultural, religious and family values supersede those of his immediate physical health. The podiatrist may have to learn to accept that empowering patients can result in the patient choosing a path which is different from that which would be regarded as suitable for solely clinical requirements. The essential characteristic of achieving concordance is the ability of the clinician to accept a viewpoint which varies from 'ideal' practice, and to be able to 'agree to differ' with their patients in a manner which is cognisant and respectful of their values.

A sustained partnership distinguishes the patient–podiatrist relationship in primary care to be different from those in other settings (Donaldson *et al.*, 1999). These relationships are different because of their more continuous, long-term nature, which fosters a familiarity between the patient and the podiatrist which in turn gives rise to a sustained partnership (Hjortdahl and Laerum, 1992; Leopold *et al.*, 1996). Such relationships are characterised by the practitioner providing support and empathy, co-participatory communication, mutual trust and an understanding of the patient as a whole person.

The importance of achieving a balance between patient autonomy and podiatrists' recommendations should not be underestimated. Since the 1990s, there has been a shift from the paternalistic approach to health care to one of mutuality and respect, independent choice and autonomy. A number of models have been proposed which describe these different approaches.

The Independent Choice Model suggests that the podiatrist's primary role in decision-making is to inform patients about their options and their relative likelihood of success. Patients are then free to make choices without the influence of the podiatrist's experience or other social constraints (Light, 1979). The Independent Choice Model is *patient-centred* and requires that the podiatrist does not bias the patient with their recommendations (Brody, 1985). The podiatrist is required to answer questions objectively, without influencing the patient, even if the patient asks for advice. Once a decision has been made, the podiatrist has to implement the podiatric aspects of that decision. There is a debate in which it is argued that patients have the right to choose inappropriate courses of treatment (Schneiderman *et al.*, 1990), and whether these should be continued indefinitely (Angell, 1991).

This model has been used within medicine, and has resulted in the doctor with values and experience becoming an impediment, rather than a resource for decision-making. This has resulted in patients often finding themselves in difficult situations without the adequate skills to make appropriate decisions (Quill and Brody, 1996).

An alternative view is provided by the Enhanced Autonomy Model, which requires the podiatrist to engage in an open dialogue with patients about therapeutic possibilities and their potential success. It also requires an exploration of the patient's values in relation to the podiatrist's values. Finally, the podiatrist offers recommendations based on *both* sets of values and experiences. This model is *relationship-centred* (both patient and podiatrist, and sometimes family members and others, are included in the decision-making process) rather than exclusively patient-centred (Pew-Fetzer, 1994). It reduces the potential for power imbalances in the relationship and reduces the possibility of a patient being manipulated or coerced by an overzealous podiatrist. Research has indicated that enhanced support of patient autonomy has been associated with better outcomes in substance abuse treatment, weight reduction and adherence to treatment regimes (Kaplan *et al.*, 1989; Ryan *et al.*, 1995; Williams *et al.*, 1996). It is this model of patient–practitioner relationships that we would encourage student podiatrists to adopt.

The Enhanced Autonomy Model involves active listening, the honest sharing of perspectives, the suspension of judgement and a genuine concern for the patient's best interests (Senge, 1990). It allows the podiatrist to support and guide their patient to use his/her knowledge, and to trust them to use that knowledge in assisting them to reach a decision.

Recommendations for enhancing patient autonomy

1. The podiatrist should understand that decisions being made by the patient have context and are based on the patient's values and experience. Common ground between the podiatrist and the patient must be sought.
2. Recommendations must consider both the clinical facts and the patient's personal experiences. While the podiatrist's perspective will be sought by the patient, the patient's values and experiences must be fed back into any recommendations that the podiatrist makes.
3. General goals should be negotiated prior to determining the technical aspects of treatment goals.
4. Where disagreements occur, and patients' wishes differ from those of the podiatrist's recommendations, then careful exploration of areas of agreement and common ground should be made first. Following this, breaking the problem down into component parts leads to a more meaningful conceptualisation and offers an opportunity of finding a way forward.
5. Final choices should be based on complete information. Both parties should be fully informed in order that common ground can be negotiated. If common ground cannot be found, then ultimately the final decision rests with the patient.
6. Podiatrists must be competent in negotiation, willing to share power in the relationship and able to demonstrate refined clinical reasoning and interviewing skills.

Motivational interviewing

Motivational interviewing (MI) is a counselling technique which was developed by two clinical psychologists, Professor William Miller and Professor Stephen Rollnick. It involves an approach which is non-judgemental, non-confrontational and non-adversarial. MI endeavours to increase a patient's awareness of the potential problems caused, consequences experienced and risks faced as a result of the behaviour in question. It aims to help clients or patients envisage a better outcome, and to become increasingly motivated to achieve it by helping patients to think differently about their behaviour and to consider what could be gained through change.

MI is considered to be both client-centred and semi-directive. Client-centred counselling was developed by the American psychologist Carl Rogers in the 1940s. It is a technique in which therapists or counsellors deliberately refrain from interpreting what their patients say but try instead to convey an attitude of unconditional positive regard in the context of a permissive, accepting, non-threatening relationship. The approach employs the techniques of clarifying, rephrasing and reflecting back the feelings or emotions that lie behind the client's words and behaviour. There is an assumption that once a person is freed from feelings of anxiety and insecurity they are capable of identifying the sources of their own emotional problems and will be able to work out their own solutions. Client-centred therapy, client-centred counselling, person-centred therapy or counselling and non-directive therapy or counselling are tangential to the traditional Rogerian counselling, whereby the therapist attempts to influence clients to consider making changes.

MI employs four basic stages:

1. **Expressing empathy**: Therapists demonstrate an understanding of the patient's perspective.
2. **Developing the patient's appreciation of discrepancies**: The therapist attempts to help clients understand the value of change by exploring the discrepancies between how they *wish* to live their lives and how they *actually* live their lives (or between deeply held values and day-to-day behaviour).
3. **Rolling with resistance**: The therapist tries to accept the client's reluctance to change as being natural rather than being pathological.
4. **Supporting self-efficacy**: The therapist needs to recognise the patient's autonomy explicitly (especially when patients choose not to change) and to help patients move towards successful change with confidence.

MI is supported by over 80 randomised clinical control trials across a range of target populations and behaviours, including substance abuse, health promotion, medical adherence and mental health issues.

MI was first used in the allied health professions in the 1990s. Since then, its efficacy has been acknowledged, particularly with patients experiencing chronic illness and long-term conditions, which require significant behavioural changes. Miller and Rollnick (2002) report favourable outcomes in the management of diabetes, cardiovascular disease, dieting, hypertension, psychosis and addictive gambling. MI works by activating patients' motivation for change and adherence to treatment. When MI is employed with patients with diabetes, those patients have been found to be more likely to continue and complete a course of treatment, participate in follow-up visits and adhere to glucose than are those patients treated by conventional approaches.

The principles that underpin MI are that:

1. Motivation to change arises from the patients and their intrinsic values, rather than being imposed by others.
2. Conventional approaches tend to have different emphases and may include unintentional coercion, or even confrontation. Such approaches may be successful in evoking behavioural change in the short term but are not sustained in the longer term.
3. The patient is encouraged to articulate the dissonance that arises from conflict provoked by different courses of action. Often, clients have not been given the opportunity to articulate such conflict or to explore the often confusing, contradictory and uniquely personal elements of their condition.

An example may be seen in the tension experienced when trying to give up smoking: 'If I stop smoking, I will feel better about myself, but I may also put on weight, which will make me feel unhappy and unattractive.' In this case, the podiatrist's role is to enable clients to explore both sides of the issue, and to guide them towards a resolution that supports long-term change.

The use of persuasion may not be the most effective way of effecting behavioural change. There is evidence that this tactic generally increases client resistance and diminishes the probability of change. Direct persuasion, aggressive confrontation and argumentation are the conceptual opposites of MI and are explicitly proscribed in this approach. MI uses slow and passive processes, which may appear laboured to those not experienced in the technique. However, evidence would suggest that more aggressive strategies, sometimes guided by a desire to 'confront client denial', push clients to make changes for which they are not ready (Miller and Rollnick, 1991; Miller et al., 1993). The podiatrist is directive in guiding the patient to examine and resolve ambivalence.

When resistance to change is encountered, this is often an indication to the podiatrist that they may need to modify motivational strategies and that the patient is not ready to undertake change.

The therapeutic relationship is more akin to a partnership or companionship rather than an expert–recipient encounter. The podiatrist respects the patient's autonomy and freedom of choice (and consequences) regarding his or her behaviour.

Summary of psychological factors

It is important to have an understanding of the sociocultural factors that will impact on patients' values and influence their decision-making strategies. Patients are encouraged to make autonomous, informed decisions about their health and treatment. Podiatrists are in a position to negotiate with patients about how desirable outcomes may be achieved and provide best advice based on a deep understanding of the patient, their needs and technical factors.

Joseph has a condition which is influenced by both his genetic make-up and by his cultural and religious beliefs. The influence of these latter factors should not be underestimated when assessing his podiatric needs and negotiating the management plan. In addition, Joseph's fears and concerns are derived from his anecdotal knowledge and his experience of diabetes in Malta with its high prevalence of amputation. These must explored with him in the context of his diet, diabetes treatment and management regime.

Implications for podiatric management

The advantages of multidisciplinary approaches to the care of a patient with a neuropathic foot ulcer cannot be overestimated. Assuring that Joseph has access to the range of services such a team offers is of paramount importance. A patient-focused treatment course must be developed, and a means of achieving it established, in order to increase the chances of a satisfactory resolution of his podiatric condition. Once achieved, the issue of prevention of reoccurrence of the ulceration must take pre-eminence over any other consideration. In order to achieve this, the podiatrist must be acutely aware of the extrinsic factors significant to the development of ulceration. Theses include cultural mores, in this instance the importance of food, celebration and *festas* in Joseph's national culture. Additional factors include occupation, and the appropriate use of off-loading methods must be considered. Success for all of these interventions and the achievement of the desired outcome are dependent on the possession of well-developed communication and listening skills.

Chapter 4

Autonomy in private practice and the need to undertake continuous professional development

Loyalty to petrified opinions never yet broke a chain or freed a human soul in this world – and never will.

Mark Twain

This chapter explores the autonomous nature of private practice. It also considers the increasing need of practitioners to undertake continuous professional development.

David Humphries qualified as a chiropodist 20 years ago before the introduction of a degree for podiatry. He trained at a small college and lived at home during his period as a student. After qualifying, he bought an established practice from a retiring practitioner, in which David still works. In the last 10 years, he has purchased one other practice in the next village, and employs two part-time practitioners and a part-time receptionist. David is married to Betty, who following some nursing experience retrained as a foot care assistant and works in his practice, where she also acts as receptionist.

David provides what he describes as 'a good traditional service', providing patients with 'what they want'. He has a busy caseload of patients who require regular appointments. David also has a large domiciliary caseload, which takes up two days of his week. Since qualifying, David has attended orthotics courses and has undertaken a course in small-business management at a local further education college. David has not been able to find time to study for a degree in podiatry, as he is very committed to charitable work locally. His practice is successful and he is rewarded by the recommendation of his patients and by the high esteem in which he is held by the local business community. Until recently, there seemed little imperative to take his studies further. However, he has started to notice that a professional journal has been publishing articles about continuous professional development (CPD). Initially, he thought this was directed towards those practitioners who had a degree. It is clear to him from the local branch of his professional body that CPD is now compulsory for all practising podiatrists. All podiatrists are now expected to accumulate a portfolio of CPD activity for each year, suitable for audit scrutiny. Professional indemnity is often linked to membership of a professional body, and this is of concern to David.

David finds this requirement daunting, and remains to be convinced that such a development is entirely necessary or, indeed, that CPD should be compulsory. However, just recently one of his part-time staff has suggested that they introduce a sports injuries and biomechanics service. This would require David to learn new skills.

The nature of private practice is very different from that of health service practice. The relationship which develops between private practitioners and their patients can be long-standing, and friendships often result. The model of the practitioner–patient relationship proposed by Szasz and Hollender (1956) and Parsons' (1951) sick role theory do not necessarily apply to private practice. Parsons suggests a set of rights and obligations for both practitioner and patient. Critics later questioned this theory because it does not explain the circumstances of chronic illness. The relationship that develops in private practice is akin to Szasz and Hollender's typology of mutual participation. Such a typology implies that the patient has a degree of power in the relationship, and therefore takes responsibility for his/her own health. This is particularly pertinent in the case of private practice, where the patient *chooses* their practitioner, and will only continue to consult them as long as they feel their needs are being met.

David is an autonomous practitioner and is in complete control of his working environment. He is confident, experienced and makes all the decisions regarding his business. He does, however, consult his employees regarding their work practices and endeavours to be flexible with and supportive of his two part-time colleagues. David is very accustomed to being in control of his life, and is both anxious and slightly affronted by the prospect of compulsory CPD. However, David realises that part of his anxiety stems from a lack of confidence in his readiness to resume study and his fear of failure.

Nevertheless, the range of patients now seen in podiatric practice has changed since David trained, and this change in case-mix is likely to present

David with a number of difficult problems. For example, it is unlikely that David will have encountered a patient such as Harriet Edmondson (Chapter 16). In addition to her psychological difficulties, Harriet is an adolescent who is likely to be demanding in ways which David will find difficult to manage. Similarly, Peter Brennan (Chapter 14) is likely to present David with issues that may challenge his personal beliefs.

The majority of patients do not attend a podiatrist for diagnosis and alleviation of their symptoms. In certain circumstances, it may not be possible to offer a cure. Patients may also seek podiatric treatment and advice for symptoms resulting from systemic illness.

Furthermore, the professional role and provision of treatment is different in private practice from practice in the state sector. Private practitioners treat anyone who seeks their services. By contrast, National Health Service practitioners may be limited by local policies and may only treat patients who meet specific access criteria and who may thus present with more complex or severe conditions.

Challenge 1: Why is David reluctant to participate in CPD?

David is currently feeling threatened for two reasons. The prospect of having to undertake CPD worries him because of the time required and because of the time that has elapsed since he last undertook any kind of formal study. Second, David feels inadequately prepared to provide a biomechanics service, as this is currently outside his scope of practice. Currently, David is avoiding addressing these issues. His habitual coping style is to ignore problems that make him feel uncomfortable or threatened rather than to address them directly.

Challenge 2: How could you avoid finding yourself in David's position?

As an undergraduate student, you have many advantages over David. For example, you will learn to develop your critical analysis skills, and to understand research methodology. These skills will enable you to keep abreast of developments in professional practice, and to employ evidence-based practice. To do this effectively, it is essential for you to understand your own learning needs and to seek appropriate post-registration education. The local branch of your professional body will offer CPD advice. In the

United Kingdom, the Health Professions Council (HPC), which is the statutory regulatory authority for podiatrists and chiropodists, agreed in 2005 the following standards for CPD:

1. The podiatrist must maintain a continuous, up-to-date and accurate record to their CPD activities.
2. The podiatrist must demonstrate that their CPD activities are a mixture of learning activities relevant to current or future practice.
3. The podiatrist must seek to ensure that their CPD has contributed to the quality of their practice and service delivery.
4. The podiatrist must seek to ensure that their CPD benefits the service user.
5. The podiatrist must present a written profile containing evidence of their CPD on request.

Podiatrists registered within the United Kingdom will be subject to regular CPD audit.

Chapter 5

Psychological and physical problems faced by middle-aged pre-menopausal women

A serious mention of menopause is usually met with uneasy silence; a sneering reference to it is usually met with relieved sniggers. Both the silence and the sniggering are pretty sure indications of taboo.

Ursula K. Le Guin

Suzi Dalton portrays some of the problems that middle-aged pre-menopausal women face. The particular psychological issues addressed are the Health Belief Model, divorce, menopause, self-esteem and factors affecting the therapeutic relationship.

Suzi is a slim, attractive woman who works as an air hostess for a large international airline. She is 48 years old, but looks slightly older than her years. She has been an air hostess since she left school and has thoroughly enjoyed the glamorous lifestyle offered by international travel. Just recently, she has begun to find it more difficult to cope with long-haul flights, and finds herself more tired than previously. She jokes that 'life begins at 40' but privately is concerned about her changed appearance and is worried about the recent irregularity of her menstrual cycle. She reports feeling more stressed than usual, and to feeling 'wound up inside'. Suzi finds herself relying more heavily on cigarettes to help get her through the difficult times. She has never had a weight problem. However, recently, she has noticed that her waist is not as slim as before. Although loath to admit it, she feels that the job was easier when she was younger, and she had more fun.

Suzi was divorced a year ago after her husband left her for a younger woman. Her manner is brusque and there is a hint of aggression in her voice. There has been an error in her appointment date and time, and she has been unpleasant and patronising to the receptionist.

Podiatric presentation

Suzi presents with painful lesser toes and a painful first metatarsalphalangeal joint. She reports that the pain is so severe that it prevents her from walking comfortably and is affecting her work. On examination, it is discovered that she has deformed toes with a number of soft-tissue lesions. Some of these are very inflamed and may be infected. In addition, there are areas of hard skin on the soles and heels of both feet. She wears high-heeled court shoes for both work and leisure; her work shoes are part of her uniform.

Factors influencing Suzi's behaviour

Suzi believes she must remain youthful in appearance in order to satisfy her employer's expectations. However, she is beginning to notice the signs of the ageing process, which causes her concern. Her tolerance to stress is reduced, and she finds she is starting to smoke more.

Suzi has low self-esteem, which may be associated with her physical appearance, which is very important to her. The slight increase in weight she has noticed is of great concern. In addition, her recent divorce has left her with feelings of rejection and inadequacy, which contribute to her reduced self-esteem. Divorce is a life event that is associated with high levels of stress. In the post-divorce period, people can experience symptoms similar to those who have been bereaved. Suzi's aggression may stem from her low self-esteem, her hormonal changes and her general unhappiness.

A number of psychosocial models have been proposed in attempts to explain people's health-related behaviours. One such model, which has been very influential in health care, is known as the Health Belief Model (Becker and Rosenstock, 1984). This model is summarised in Figure 5.1.

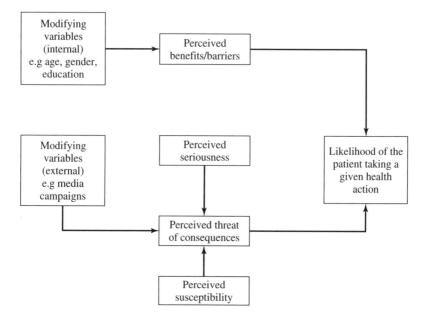

Figure 5.1 The Health Belief Model. (*Source:* Adapted from Becker and Rosenstock, 1984.)

The major components of the model are as follows:

Demographic factors

Suzi's beliefs are influenced by her age, gender and occupation. She works in an industry in which physical appearance, youth and attractiveness are considered important attributes.

Susceptibility

The likelihood of an individual performing any given behaviour is in part determined by how susceptible they believe they are to any outcome that may be associated with that behaviour. In Suzi's case, the likelihood of her changing her footwear (the probable cause of her pain) depends in part on her beliefs regarding the relation between fashion shoes and the development of her foot condition.

Severity

Severity refers to the extent to which Suzi believes that hallux valgus is a serious condition.

Benefits and costs

These factors combine to form Suzi's perception of the threat to her foot health, and it is on this perception, together with the other factors shown in Figure 5.1, that Suzi will base decision about changing her footwear. The model proposes that Suzi will weigh up the various benefits and costs of her taking any particular course of action (or of taking no action). From Suzi's perspective, the benefits of wearing fashionable shoes may outweigh the costs of her developing hallux valgus.

Challenge 1: What are the bio-psychosocial risk factors for Suzi?

The first issue to consider is the ageing process. Bond and Colman (1990) note that there is an inherent sexism attached to processes of ageing. Whilst changes in physical appearance, such as greying hair, are seen as signs of increasing maturity in men, they are viewed as a waning of femininity in women. Suzi may be particularly vulnerable in this respect because of her occupation and the value she attaches to her physical appearance.

A second important issue for Suzi is the prospect of the menopause, which usually commences in the fifth decade of life. Symptoms of the menopause include hot flushes and night sweats. It is also sometimes associated with low self-esteem, irritability and reduced libido. Other changes which occur at a similar time to the menopause may also impact on social identity and self-esteem. For example, children leaving home, divorce and elderly parents becoming dependent may result in considerable psychological upheaval. Conversely, this period may be accompanied by a reappraisal of values and ambitions, which may result in greater contentment.

In addition to the psychological and physical changes that accompany the menopause, Suzi will have to consider the effects of osteoporosis. Osteoporosis is the commonest metabolic disease of bone and is most frequently found in women following the menopause. While the effects of osteoporosis are systemic, manifestations may also be found in the feet. Symptoms include pain, and sufferers are more susceptible to fractures. Smoking significantly increases the risk of developing osteoporosis.

On average, women who smoke reach the menopause up to two years earlier than do women who are non-smokers. This is partly because chemicals in cigarette smoke reduce levels of oestrogen in the blood. Smoking also constricts blood vessels, which leads to the exacerbation of symptoms such as hot flushes.

In Suzi's case, smoking and being menopausal combine in such a way that the sum is greater than a simple combination of the effects of these two factors. This effect is known as *synergy*.

The menopause is also a time that can be associated with an increase in weight. An increase in weight and change in body size and shape may have a negative effect on Suzi's self-image and self-esteem. In addition, it may increase the pain and discomfort she feels in her feet.

Self-esteem is concerned with how worthwhile and confident individuals feel about themselves. Self-esteem is a component of a complex self-system (Harter, 1988a, 1988b) that is composed of a number of components, such as academic achievement, social acceptance, physical appearance and athletic ability. It may be viewed as either high or low depending on an individual's interpretation of their abilities. It is also possible to have low scores for one component and still feel generally good about oneself. It is suggested that individuals have high self-esteem when the attributes that they like about themselves outweigh those that they dislike. This balance may be altered by life events. In the case of significant events, such as divorce, self-esteem may be decreased for extended periods (Harter, 1985). In addition, transitional life stages may also exert a negative effect on self-esteem. Such episodes are described as *midlife crises* (Simmons *et al.*, 1983). The effect of conflict between an individual's notions about their ideal self and observations of their actual self may result in chronic anxiety or depression (Rogers, 1951).

Suzi's self-esteem is likely to be affected by her recent divorce (Figure 5.2). Divorce is acknowledged to be a highly disruptive life event, the effects of which can range from devastation to relief (Diedrick, 1991). Divorce adjustment has generally been measured in terms of self-esteem. Some

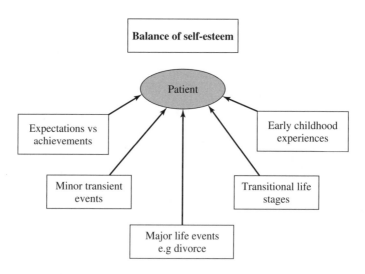

Figure 5.2 Components of self-esteem. (*Source:* Adapted from Russell, 1999, with permission of Routledge.)

research suggests that self-esteem works as a type of defence mechanism (Cast and Burke, 2002). It can be built up but also lost, particularly as it is responsive to change in social circumstances. When individuals are unable to confirm their identities, the self-esteem produced by previous successful efforts at self-verification buffers or protects individuals from the distress associated with a lack of self-verification (when self-verification processes are disrupted), thereby preserving threatened structural arrangements (Burke, 1991). In protecting the self against distress while the situation is 'resolved' (Thoits, 1994), however, self-esteem is used up or diminished. Thus, self-esteem is analogous to a reservoir of energy. Like any other resource, self-esteem can be built up, but when used it is lost.

Divorce is a common trigger to suffering depression. Depression is characterised by sadness, low self-esteem, disturbed sleep patterns and weight gain or loss. Podiatrists need to be aware of the increase in the divorce rate, which will inevitably bring them into contact with patients suffering the psychological effects of separation and divorce.

Finally, Suzi needs to consider that her footwear may be contributing to the painful and infected lesions that she presents with between her toes. One of the consequences of wearing inappropriate footwear may be a delay in the resolution of Suzi's infection.

Challenge 2: Convince Suzi of the benefits of change

You are concerned about the condition of Suzi's feet, and in particular the possible infection of her toes. For any of your treatment options to be successful, Suzi must begin to wear more sensible footwear. Therefore, your first priority is to convince her that the benefits of change outweigh any disadvantages.

How to assist your patient to change

Identify the barriers to communication

In Suzi's case, these barriers may consist of depression, stress, fear and anger. The podiatrist should listen, be empathetic and try to reach a point of common agreement. It is certainly essential to keep calm and avoid any confrontation. It is important to remain detached, making it clear that no personal criticism is implied in the conversation. Confrontation may lead to a heightened sense of arousal.

If Suzi indicates that she is considering making a formal complaint, the podiatrist should always agree to investigate the nature of her complaint. It is also very important to be familiar with the complaints procedure. It is possible that an error in the appointment system occurred, and the podiatrist must apologise if this is the case. If no error has occurred, then it is important to adopt an empathetic neutral approach.

Health care professionals also rely on non-verbal behaviour to aid communication. Empathy can be conveyed using appropriate non-verbal skills; facial expressions, eye contact, touch and proximity can help break down communication barriers. The use of appropriate volume, tone and pitch in speech can also defuse difficult communication situations effectively.

Suzi should be given the space and opportunity to articulate her problems and her perception of them. At the outset, Suzi may only talk about the superficial and immediate problems associated with her appointment. However, as trust becomes established, Suzi may become more confident in the relationship and may be ready to discuss her more personal problems.

Once Suzi's agenda has been established, communication can progress. There may be occasions when the podiatrist and the patient have different expectations, for example the patient's expectations may be unrealistic. Conversely, the podiatrist may expect the patient to achieve more than is reasonable. It is therefore helpful during this phase to encourage the patient to discuss her treatment and prognosis expectations, and to negotiate realistic and achievable goals.

In the literature, *communication* is generally considered under the headings of *verbal communication* and *non-verbal behaviour*. Verbal communication is concerned with the spoken language. Language used when engaging in professional conversations should not be complicated by jargon, and the delivery of information should be in manageable units that are clearly understood by the patient. Some useful techniques include using phrases such as: 'What I am going to tell you now is important' or 'You need to listen carefully to what I am about to say', which alert the patient to the fact that what they are about to hear must be listened to and understood. Phrases such as this herald important information. Questioning styles may be open, allowing the respondent to elaborate on their thoughts, feelings and concerns, much like the counselling style (McLoughlin, 1996). Closed questions are best used to find out facts and which only require simple yes/no responses, for example a closed question could be: 'Is ibuprofen the only NSAID you take?' An open question, for example, could be: 'What medication are you currently taking?' If a communication request is made, then even more information may be elicited, for example: 'Tell me about the medication you are currently taking.'

If the patient has difficulty understanding English, arrangements should be made for an interpreter to be present. The use of interpreters is discussed in Chapter 9.

Non-verbal behaviour is often described as *paralinguistics*, and concerns pace, tone, pitch, volume, dialect and pauses. It focuses on the way in which information is delivered, rather than what is actually said (Dickson *et al.*, 1997). Utterances may sometimes replace words to provide feedback, and regulate the speed at which a conversation occurs. Other components of non-verbal behaviour include touch, posture, position, gestures, facial expression and personal proximity.

Touch is an important part of communication for the podiatrist. Professional touch is when the podiatrist touches the patient in order to carry out treatment, for example in the assessment of pulses, range of joint motion and the reduction of corns and calluses. Therapeutic touch can be regarded as touch through which the therapeutic relationship is built, for example shaking hands or a sympathetic touch of the arm. It has been suggested that the position adopted by the podiatrist has a profound effect on the relationship that podiatrists develop with their patients (Mandy, P., 2000).

Gestures and facial expression may be used to encourage or discourage engagement in communication. Eye contact is a method that can be used to control communication and terminate it at an appropriate juncture (Dickson *et al.*, 1997).

Gaze is a term that refers to a person's behaviour while *looking*. Gaze is an important function to the gathering of information. Although gaze avoidance deprives us of valuable information about how others respond, this may be normative in some cultures and in certain situations. Gaze avoidance may occur because of deference to the speaker, fear of revealing feelings or fear of negative feedback. It is also used to express feelings, intentions and attitudes. One of the most important functions of gaze is to regulate the flow of a conversation, and we all have a rough-and-ready idea of what amount of gaze is normal. Normally, we look at a person when we are listening to them. We look away when we are speaking, glancing at the listener every so often to ensure that they've not fallen asleep and to gain feedback as to the effect our message is having. There is therefore a natural imbalance in the amount of gaze. Argyle (1990) suggests that, normally, listeners actively gaze for about 70% of the communication, while the figure is 40% of the communication for speakers. Anything departing much from these norms will be perceived as abnormal.

Posture and positioning are also important elements of non-verbal communication. Positioning is an interesting component and one that cannot be changed easily for the podiatrist. Traditionally, the podiatrist will sit facing the patient's feet, which will be positioned at a comfortable height for treatment. This will often result in the patient being positioned above the podiatrist. It has been suggested (Mandy, P., 2000) that such positioning may be subconsciously indicative of a subservient role.

The rules for proximity vary according to culture and ethnic groups. There are, however, established distance zones (ranging from intimate, to personal, social and public) that can be generally applied to situations. An intimate distance for love-making and comforting can range from six to

18 inches. Personal distance ranges from 18 inches to four feet and distances in a social setting can range from four to seven feet at the near phase and seven to 12 feet at the far phase. In public, distances are typically greater, from 12 to 25 feet or more. Preferences for spacing will influence where the people sit or stand (Argyle, 1990).

Identify the factors that will enable you to establish a therapeutic relationship

The podiatrist needs to make Suzi sufficiently comfortable within the relationship to discuss sensitive material that may affect her care. Frequently, patients are unaware of the impact that apparently unrelated factors can have on their foot health. For example, Suzi may not acknowledge that her menopause may be related to the development of hard skin on her heels and soles of her feet. Similarly, she may not associate the lesions on her toes with pressure and friction from footwear. In order to achieve a satisfactory relationship, the podiatrist should exhibit a warm, non-judgemental, open and caring approach. The podiatrist must actively *listen* to the patient.

As long ago as 1956, Szasz and Hollender described a model in which different typologies of relationships may be observed. *Active/passive typology* is a term used to describe circumstances in which the therapist is the active participant and the patient is solely a passive recipient of treatment. An example of this would be the comatose patient in the Emergency Department who is attended to by the medical team. This typology is not usually encountered in podiatric practice.

In Szasz and Hollender's (1956) Guidance/Co-operative typology, it is assumed that the podiatrist has access to knowledge and information that would make him/her equipped to offer advice and guidance, having taken the patient's wishes into account. In this typology, the podiatrist continues to dominate the question-and-answer sessions.

In the Mutual Participation typology, Szasz and Hollender (1956) propose that the consultation is characterised by a negotiation between both parties. Patients acknowledge the skills and expertise of the podiatrist, while retaining their right to decide on their own treatment.

In certain circumstances, Szasz and Hollender (1956) suggest a further typology, which they call Passive/Active. This situation exists when the patient is in possession of all the relevant facts concerning their condition, understands the treatment that is necessary and simply uses the podiatrist to provide it. Patients increasingly have access to relevant information, using resources such as the Internet, and are providing health care professionals with more challenging interactions (Neuberger, 2000). Some practitioners may find this increasing patient autonomy difficult to deal with because it represents a shift of power within the relationship, a shift which may make the podiatrist feel that their position is being threatened.

The concept of the active patient has developed since the mid-1980s as a result of a general move towards a more consumerist society (Wiles and Higgins, 1996). However, the notion of consumerism in medicine is complicated since it presumes that the patient is in a position to make an informed choice. However, within state-provided health care, there is in fact little choice available. Morgan (1991) proposes that there are four types of doctor–patient relationship, based upon the degree of control exercised by the doctor and the patient. He suggests that challenges to medical authority have resulted in the doctor–patient relationship moving in the direction of mutuality, where permitted, in state-provided health care.

May *et al.* (2003) suggest that patients are now encouraged to think of themselves as active consumers of health rather than passive recipients. Gafaranga and Britten (2003) endorse this notion of mutuality and have explored the ways in which it may be achieved. Using an ethnomethodological approach, and conversation analysis, they propose the concept of *alignment* as a central tenet of communication. Patients and practitioners are said to be *aligned* if they share an understanding of the *here and now situation*. Alignment is constructed step by step; however, if misalignment occurs, it tends to happen at the beginning of a consultation, and if this is the case concordance is harder to achieve.

Such passivity has led historically to the notion of compliance. Much literature exists concerning the problems of the 'non-compliance' of patients with prescribed treatment programmes. Since the 1990s, the term *compliance* has been replaced with *adherence*, which, while acknowledging a contribution towards treatment on the part of the patient other than through simply obeying medical authority, still fails to fully embrace the notion of the patient as an active contributor to their treatment and ultimate well-being (Gafaranga and Britten, 2003). For this reason, the term *concordance* is increasingly being used to describe the way in which a patient reacts to the advice and information offered by a practitioner. Many texts continue to use the terms adherence and compliance synonymously. The term concordance requires an understanding of the patient's health beliefs, and an attempt to make them congruent with a course of action that will result in the maximum health gain. In Suzi's case, this will involve her choosing more appropriate footwear, using recommended medications and wearing appropriate orthotics.

Achieving concordance requires the podiatrist to be able to provide the necessary information in a way that is credible, understandable and acceptable to the patient. This may be achieved by developing communication skills, and by the provision of written information that is presented in short sentences using uncomplicated language. The use of readability indices can help in ensuring that the message will be understood by potential readers. Readability indices are readily available on most personal computers.

In addition, when designing a treatment plan, the patient and podiatrist should work together to provide an achievable regimen with realistic targets and timeframes. Reinforcement should be built into the plan to assist in the achievement of targets and goals. When there is a complex regimen, it is often useful to suggest ways in which tasks may be simplified. If the patient can incorporate a task into their everyday life, it is more likely that they will undertake it, for example encouraging a patient to apply foot cream after bathing will turn the task into a routine (Figure 5.3).

Alder (1999) suggests that the process of making decisions does not always rely on logic but on perceived probabilities. The rules for working with probabilities are called *heuristics*, which can have potential biases (Alder, 1999). We shall now investigate heuristics, as it pertains to Suzi's case.

The *availability heuristic* is a judgement based on available information about the subject of interest. Suzi may, for example, expect that her menopause is likely to happen during her fifties.

The *representative heuristic* is a judgement based on information that is typical for a given group of people. Thus, if Suzi were to miss her period

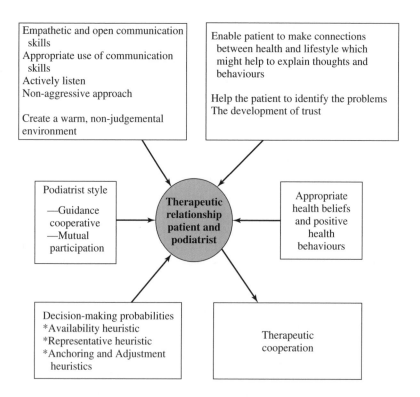

Figure 5.3 Factors affecting the therapeutic relationship

in her fifties, she might assume that she was menopausal, but during her twenties she would have suspected pregnancy.

Anchoring and *adjustment heuristics* enable people to make judgements from a given starting point. For example, missing a period at the age of 47 may lead Suzi to think that she was experiencing her menopause earlier than her availability heuristic would suggest.

Achievement of therapeutic cooperation

It is necessary to understand why Suzi insists on wearing court shoes. Often, patients will insist that shoes which are potentially damaging to their feet are actually quite comfortable. The podiatrist will need to use skilled questioning in order to elicit from Suzi when she experiences pain, and what she does to relieve that pain.

It is important that Suzi recognise the role her shoes have in causing her symptoms, and that she understands that other footwear may be more appropriate. It may be helpful to suggest that being more comfortable may influence her work performance positively and improve her general sense of well-being. At this point, Suzi may be more receptive to advice, and may be more likely to consider a change in the style of her shoes. In addition, she will need information to help her to make informed choices.

If Suzi is unwilling to change her shoe style whilst at work, it may be possible to negotiate that she wears comfortable, well-fitting shoes during her leisure time. Such a compromise can often lead to full concordance with the treatment plan at a later date.

Summary of important health psychology

Communication is the key factor when treating patients such as Suzi. The use of appropriate communication skills will enable the successful development of the therapeutic relationship. An understanding and application of the Health Belief Model will assist the podiatrist in helping Suzi change her foot health behaviour. In addition, a better understanding of the more general psychological and physiological factors which influence Suzi's current behaviour will be valuable in this process. In particular, podiatrists should be aware of the impact that menopausal symptoms can have on their patients' physical and psychological well-being.

Implications for podiatric management

It is likely that after one or two assessment visits to the podiatrist Suzi will find it difficult to accommodate the behavioural change which has been advised, in particular smoking cessation and changes to footwear. In order to alleviate immediate symptoms and to prevent further deterioration, Suzi will need to acknowledge that a change to her footwear is required, at least for the majority of the time. Increasingly in modern podiatric practice, orthotic devices are becoming available that can be used in less than optimum footwear. It is the job of the podiatrist to discuss all available treatment methods, what can reasonably be expected as an outcome of each method and to rely on the patient to make appropriate judgements. However, it is certainly incumbent on the podiatrist to ensure that they have offered all of the information available, including a robust evaluation of the risks associated with each option, in order that the patient can make informed choices. The use of motivational interviewing (Chapter 3) would facilitate such a negotiation.

Chapter 6

Symptoms of a work-related injury

Real success is finding your lifework in the work that you love.
David McCullough

Jayne Ellis is a senior podiatrist who has been qualified for five years. During this time, she has worked for three health care providers in order to gain experience and enable her to be promoted to a senior grade with some management responsibility. Professionally, Jayne feels as if she has developed a good knowledge and expertise in her practice and feels competent in her daily work. She has paid off her student loan and has been able to finance herself through a part-time master's degree course. She felt she needed to do this if she wished to be promoted again but also because she is beginning to feel that she should stimulate her brain again with more academic work.

Factors influencing Jayne's behaviour

Jayne is beginning to feel that her current employer is not meeting her needs. The prospect of promotion is minimal, as the management hierarchy to which she subscribes is dominated by other health professionals who have been in post for several years and who do not appear to wish to move area or are unlikely to be promoted. Jayne believes she will have to move areas if she is to achieve the promotion that she requires, but is reluctant to do this because she has just purchased her first flat and is settled near friends and family. She is disappointed that she is beginning to develop feelings of boredom and frustration within her work, and is losing the sense of achievement that she once felt. The degree course gave her a renewed enthusiasm and desire to undertake more research within her clinical practice. However, since completing her studies, there has been a period of rationalisation within her department, which has resulted in an increased caseload for the staff that remain. Jayne currently feels that any hope of undertaking research within the clinical environment has been lost and she is left with the increasing feelings of frustration and despondency.

In addition to this, Jayne has noticed that she has begun to experience wrist pain towards the end of the clinical sessions, particularly when she has had extra patients to see. She keeps a packet of ibuprofen in her trolley drawer and takes a couple when the pain gets too bad.

Challenge 1: What is the cause of Jayne's dissatisfaction with her daily work?

A review of the literature suggests that the nature and scope of professional practice has not changed, to any large extent, even though the pre- and post-registration curriculum has expanded. In 1993, Merriman suggested that, traditionally, the nature of podiatric practice incorporated palliative type treatments aimed at keeping patients ambulatory, independent and active. Nearly a decade later, in 2001, a study by Macdonald and Capewell reported that podiatrists were frustrated by undertaking low-skilled tasks which could be performed by health care assistants or voluntary groups. A year later, further work by Farndon et al. evaluated the professional role of the podiatrist in the new millennium. The results concurred with the earlier studies and suggested that the most frequent area of clinical practice involved simple professional techniques which did not professionally challenge practitioners. Moreover, the conclusions reported by Farndon et al. suggested that the nature of the work had not changed since 1993, when Merriman first reviewed the scope of professional podiatric practice. Farndon et al. (2002) further suggested that, following the publication of The NHS Plan (Department of Health, 2000), core skills would be identified and practice defined in the hope that this would engender a shift from the traditionally described palliative model to a more curative model. It was anticipated that a shift in service delivery would result in podiatrists being able to draw on the complete range of their professional skills.

In 2007, Mandy et al. reported a study which explored the patterns of employment of podiatrists, from newly qualified to those who had been qualified for five years. One of the most notable findings from this study was the attrition rate for podiatry, which increased the longer podiatrists were qualified. Reasons for leaving the profession included professional dissatisfaction, poor financial remuneration and the need to change career. Those members that were still within the profession similarly reported work stress and themes of frustration with the lack of professional status, which were equitable to those reported by Jenny Fraser in Chapter 2.

However, some had used promotional opportunities to be able to specialise in certain areas, which helped to reduce such feelings. Alternatively, some had chosen to combine their state health practice with private practice. Private practice was perceived to provide better financial remuneration, a more flexible working environment, improved pension provision and greater flexibility within the work environment. These positive attributes were predominantly seen as important for female members of the profession, particularly when considering taking career breaks to have children.

Challenge 2: What are the implications of Jayne's wrist pain?

The most commonly reported type of work-related illness in the United Kingdom is work-related musculoskeletal disorder (WRMD) (Health and Safety Executive, 2007). In total, 4.7 million working days (full-day equivalent) were lost in 2004/05 through musculoskeletal disorders, mainly affecting the upper limbs or neck and caused or made worse by work. On average, people suffering from work-related upper-limb disorders (WRULDs) took 21.7 days off work in 2004/5. This equates to an annual loss of 0.2 days per worker.

Moreover, results from the latest survey of self-reported work-related illness indicate that in 2005/06 an estimated prevalence of 374 000 people in Great Britain suffered, in their opinion, from a musculoskeletal disorder mainly affecting the upper limbs or neck that was caused or made worse by their current or past work. This equates to 870 per 100 000 people (0.87%) who have ever worked in Great Britain.

The most frequently reported diagnostic site for both males and females affected with upper-limb disorders were the hands, wrist and arms, with health care workers being identified as an industry with one of the highest prevalence rates of this kind of work-related illness (Health and Safety Executive, 2007). Factors that contribute to the aetiology of WRMDs include repetitive action, high force exertion and fatigue. Psychosocial factors, such as job control and interpersonal relationships, have also been identified as playing a role (Carayon *et al.*, 1999; Muggleton *et al.*, 1999; Halford and Cohen, 2003).

Birtles and Leah (2006) report that podiatrists are particularly predisposed to musculoskeletal disorders. Within this group, lower-back pain is the most commonly reported disorder (71%), followed by shoulder problems (31%) and finally wrist pain (27%). The risk factors associated with the work of a podiatrist include:

- compromised postures, where joints of the body are held at the extreme of ranges of motion
- static body postures, where parts of the body are held in the same posture for extended periods
- high-risk postures local to the upper body, such as flexion or rotation of the wrist, or prolonged elevation of the wrist or shoulder while the podiatrist reaches or stoops to access parts of the patient's foot to apply treatment
- treatments often involving repetitive applications of force that increase the risk of injury, such as using nail nippers.

A particular risk factor for work-related upper-extremity disorder is prolonged static pressure. Pheasant (1994) developed a model of pathogenesis (Figure 6.1) which identified static pressure as being a particular risk factor for upper-limb WRMDs and in particular carpal tunnel syndrome, tendonitis and neurovascular disorders such as Raynaud's syndrome. Symptoms include numbness, aching, oedema, pain and loss of function (Lowe and Freivalds, 1999). Pain can manifest in a number of ways, including nocturnal tingling, gradual numbness, prickling and dull aching (Treaster and Burr, 2004).

There are only three reported studies of WRMDs in the podiatry literature (Piggott, 1991; Shaw et al., 2001; Layzell, 2004). Moreover, Layzell's study (2004) is the only one to explore upper-limb disorders and to suggest podiatry-specific factors that have the potential to put practitioners at risk. These include:

- repetition of tasks, e.g. fine-hand movements used in debridement or corn enucleation
- poor maintenance of instruments, e.g. blunting of scissors and nippers may result in the podiatrist requiring greater force to operate
- static posture, whereby the practitioner adopts an awkward or uncomfortable position. Tasks such as skin debridement or corn enucleation may cause pain in the shoulders and upper limbs.

Other common factors include the number of patients treated, the length of the working day, the nature of the patients' treatments and the number of breaks within a working day.

Poor maintenance of equipment is also an important issue. Equipment that is routinely sterilised through a central sterilisation services department (CSSD) will become blunt more quickly than if bench-top sterilizers are used. Instrument technique and appropriately sized instruments are

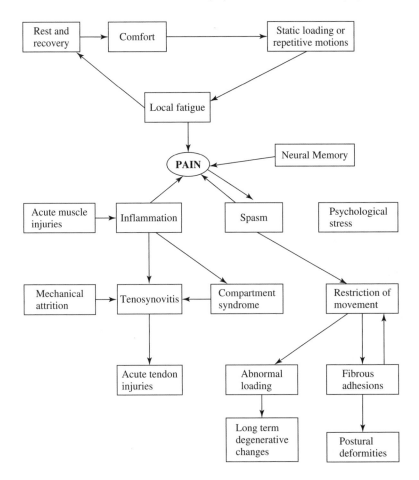

Figure 6.1 Pheasant's proposed model of the pathogenesis of WRMDs

also issues that should be considered. Halford and Birch (2005) suggest that inappropriate instrumentation technique in addition to poor mainte-nance are influential in the development of WRMD and that it is a dual responsibility between the employee and manager to ensure safe working practices.

Jayne is also responsible for a domiciliary caseload, which she undertakes once a week. She has noticed that her wrist pain is particularly worse after a day of domiciliary visits.

Domiciliary treatment can be particularly challenging for podiatrists, because they are often expected to work in environments that maybe unsuitable. Jayne has often been forced to sit on a stool, or squat on the floor, whilst the patient sits on a sofa to undergo treatment. The lighting is often inappropriate and she has struggled to cope. In addition to this, her instruments are stored in a domiciliary case into which she has to continually reach. Domiciliary visits will also have a significant number of work-related psychosocial risks factors. For example, Jayne visits a lonely mentally ill patient who lives on the seventh floor of a block of flats in which the lift is invariably out of order.

The link between psychosocial issues, such as increased attentional demands, lack of support and paced work set by a third party, have been linked to the increased prevalence of WRMDs (Devereux *et al.*, 1999). The Health and Safety Executive research and guidance discloses six key areas of work, which, if not correctly managed, are associated with poor health and well-being. These include:

- **demands**: workload, work pattern and work environment
- **control**: how much control Jayne has over her work
- **support**: including encouragement, sponsorship and resources provided by the organisation, line management and colleagues
- **relationship**: includes promoting positive working to avoid conflict and dealing with unacceptable behaviour
- **role**: whether employees understand their role within the organisation and whether the organisation ensures that the person does not have conflicting roles
- **change**: how organisational change (large or small) is managed and communicated within the organisation.

The presence of these psychosocial risk factors will impact on the musculoskeletal well-being of podiatrists, with individual variation. Some podiatrists will feel comfortable with their multifaceted jobs, whereas for others this will be a source of regular or constant stress.

There are psychobiological mechanisms that make a connection between WRMDs and work stress plausible (Carayon *et al.*, 1999). Psychological stress can lead to increased physiological susceptibility, which in turn can affect hormonal, circulatory and respiratory responses. Furthermore, it can also affect attitudes, motivation and behaviours towards work and actions, which can increase the risk of WRMD. Psychosocial work factors are those that affect employees emotionally and result in stress and strain (Hagberg, 1992). The quality and intensity of the emotion and its effect on physiological and behavioural changes are dependent upon the present or anticipated significance of the interaction with the environment and the threat to that person's security and safety. Psychosocial work factors such as quantity and quality of work, lack of job control and job future ambiguity can all result in the stress experience, which in turn can affect an individual's motivation towards work.

Summary of important health psychology

Work organisation factors and job stress play an important role in the development of WRMDs, in addition to traditional ergonomic risk factors, such as repetition, force and posture. Moreover, organisational and ergonomic factors interact or are related to each other, which in turn contributes to the development of WRMDs. Thus, in order to understand this complex phenomenon more deeply, it is important to examine physical, ergonomic and psychosocial work factors in the context of the work organisation.

Implications for podiatric management

The health and safety of staff is a responsibility for all employers and for those who are self-employed. There are a number of statutory requirements and regulations that apply which can be accessed on the Health and Safety Executive's website (http://www.hse.gov.uk). The prevention of WRMDs is important to reduce suffering and to avoid costly employment tribunals and litigation. When staff experience WRMDs and stress-related disorders, which in turn result in sick leave, there is a knock-on effect for those remaining staff who are providing cover. In turn, these staff may then experience occupational stress, which can impact on the morale of the entire team.

It should be seen as the responsibility of all podiatrists to reflect on their own health and safety and to access appropriate resources to reduce the risks as much as possible. Those managing services should move health and safety and occupational health to the centre of organisational structures when planning service delivery.

Chapter 7

Health decision-making based on the theory of reasoned action

We are responsible for actions performed in response to circumstances for which we are not responsible.

Allan Massie

The theory of reasoned action is used to explain how Charles Walters makes decisions about his health. The sick role, self-help groups and retirement are also explored.

Charles is 52-year-old ex-policeman who has retired early on medical grounds. In the past five years, he has developed maturity onset diabetes, which he has been unable to control by modification of his diet, and therefore has to take tablets. He is overweight and does not undertake any exercise. Charles had worked for the police force since leaving school at 16 years of age. He was committed to his chosen career and it fulfilled his life. He is not married, and because of his lifelong commitment to his work has found the transition into early retirement difficult. He has few interests outside of work and has not had time to develop any social activities. He recognises that his diabetes has got worse and admits that he finds it difficult to control his diet, and he thinks he is too old to start any sport.

Charles knows that he is eligible for podiatry treatment because of his diabetes.

He presents with only minor podiatric problems, but he attends the podiatry clinic regularly for assessment and monitoring. As part of the multiprofessional team that is involved in diabetic care, the podiatrist will not only assess his neurological and vascular status but also be concerned with preventing the development of diabetic complications.

Factors influencing Charles's behaviour

Charles has good intentions regarding his diabetes, but, in his words, he 'enjoys his food'. However, he also believes that the services provided by the 'specialist' health care workers will be more influential in controlling his diabetes better, because 'they are the professionals'. As a result, he has become quite dependent on all the people in the clinics he has to attend. Charles's diet is not very well controlled, and it is important that the podiatrist understands how Charles makes choices about what he eats.

A number of theories have been proposed which try to explain how people make health-related decisions. These models are known collectively as *social cognition models*, and many applications are noted in the health psychology literature. One of the most important of these is the Theory of Reasoned Action (Fishbein and Ajzen, 1975; Figure 7.1).

In this case, Charles's *behavioural beliefs* may include:

- Eating a healthy diet will help reduce the complications of my diabetes.
- Eating a healthy diet will help me lose weight.
- Eating a healthy diet will improve my ability to heal.

All the *outcome evaluations* corresponding to these beliefs are likely to be *positive*. Conversely, Charles's behavioural beliefs may also include:

- A healthy diet is boring.
- Being unable to drink with my friends restricts my social life.
- I'd have to give up all the things I like if I eat a healthy diet.

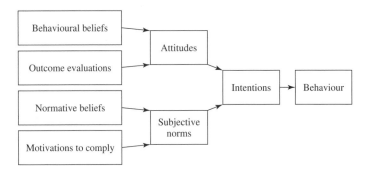

Figure 7.1 The Theory of Reasoned Action. (*Source:* Adapted from Fishbein and Ajzen, 1975, after Sutton, 1989. © John Wiley & Sons. Reproduced with permission.)

All the *outcome evaluations* corresponding to these beliefs are likely to be *negative*.

These conflicting behavioural beliefs and evaluations combine to produce Charles's *attitudes* to changing his diet.

Charles *normative beliefs* concerning eating a healthy diet may include:

■ My specialists think that improving my diet would help my diabetes.
■ The people managing my treatment are experts in diabetes.

Charles's *motivations* to comply may include:

■ I want to please the specialists who are looking after me.
■ Experts know best, so I'll try really hard to diet.

However, Charles's *normative beliefs* concerning eating a healthy diet may also include:

■ Being amongst my old work mates is more important than what doctors tell you.

In this case, Charles's *motivations* to comply may include:

■ I'm not going to be told what to do by so-called experts.

These conflicting normative beliefs and motivations combine to produce Charles's *subjective norms* in relation to changing his diet. Charles's behavioural beliefs and subjective norms in turn combine to influence his *intention* to either change his diet or continue his previous pattern of eating.

If the podiatrist can influence Charles's beliefs and thus his attitudes towards changing his diet, this might increase the likelihood of changing his intentions towards changing his diet. Such influence is dependent on the quality of the therapeutic relationship that is formed between the podiatrist, Charles and the diabetic team. The nature and importance of the therapeutic relationship is described in Chapter 4.

A variant of the Theory of Reasoned Action is the Theory of Planned Behaviour (Ajzen and Madden, 1986; Figure 7.2), which has attracted considerable attention. In addition to the components of the Theory of Reasoned Action a further element is included which is known as *perceived behavioural control*. This component is a direct measure of the degree of control that individuals feel they have over the behaviour in question. Perceived behavioural control is an important addition to the model,

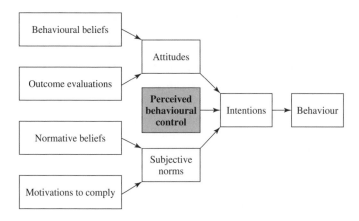

Figure 7.2 The Theory of Planned Behaviour. (*Source:* Adapted from Ajzen and Madden, 1986, after Sutton 1989. © John Wiley & Sons. Reproduced with permission.)

particularly in the case of behaviours that contain an addictive component, for example smoking, drinking or other drug use.

However, it is important to note that there is discussion as to the discrete nature of perceived behavioural control in the manner proposed by Ajzen and Madden. No agreed standards are available for measuring the components of the model, and while some authors have found self-efficacy (a concept which many consider to be synonymous with perceived behavioural control) to significantly predict behavioural intentions in the manner proposed by the Theory of Planned Behaviour (Terry and O'Leary, 1995) other authors have not (Povey *et al.*, 2000).

Nevertheless, for many years, the Theory of Planned Behaviour has been used in attempts to explain a wide range of health-related behaviours. Applications include studies of cigarette smoking, alcohol and drug use, exercise behaviour, concordance with medical treatments and dietary advice. However, the models such as the Theory of Reasoned Action and Theory of Planned Behaviour have a number of shortcomings, which have become widely recognised amongst health psychologists (for example Roberts *et al.*, 2001). Notably, the models assume that people act in a logical and rational way, which many consider to be unrealistic. Second, while subjective norms and attitudes predict intentions quite well in statistical analyses, the models' overall ability to predict actual behaviour is limited. Perhaps most importantly, such models fail to appreciate the complexity of the social context in which most health-related behaviours are located.

Challenge 1: Consider what other factors may be important in influencing Charles's behaviour that are not included within the theory of reasoned action and theory of planned behaviour models

The *sick role* was a concept introduced by Parsons in 1951. Parsons defined *health* as a 'state of optimum capacity for effective role performance'. Conversely, illness is a generalised disturbance of this state. Where role capacity is affected by illness, the individual is given a status and role in society, that of the *sick person*. The sick role is characterised by rights and obligations for both the sick person and the health practitioner who treats them. There are four main features of the sick role:

1. The sick person is exempt from the performance of their social duties. This exemption requires validation by others, especially medical practitioners, who have been given the power to determine whether a person is sick or not.
2. The sick person is not held responsible for their state of health. Therefore, the sick person cannot be asked to 'pull themselves together and get better'.
3. The sick person is obliged to give up the right to engage in activities normally undertaken by healthy people. If a person suffering from a heavy cold has entered the sick role and taken a day off from work they are then not entitled, according to the sick role, to go out that same evening to attend a social event.
4. The sick are obliged to seek qualified help where appropriate and to follow the advice of a qualified practitioner.

Charles is happy to accept some of the rights of the sick role but few of the obligations.

The term *diabetes mellitus* describes a metabolic disorder of multiple aetiology characterised by chronic hyperglycaemia with disturbances of carbohydrate, fat and protein metabolism resulting from defects in insulin secretion or insulin action, or both (World Health Organization, 1999). The effects of diabetes mellitus include long-term damage to and the dysfunction and failure of various organs.

The long-term effects of diabetes mellitus include the progressive development of the specific complications of retinopathy, with potential blindness; nephropathy, which may lead to renal failure; and/or neuropathy, with its risk of foot ulcers, amputation, Charcot's joints; and features of autonomic dysfunction, including sexual dysfunction. People with diabetes are at increased risk of cardiovascular, peripheral vascular and cerebrovascular disease.

Diabetes mellitus can be classified into two types. Type 1 encompasses the majority of cases that are primarily due to pancreatic islet beta-cell destruction and are prone to ketoacidosis. Type 1 includes those cases attributable to an autoimmune process, as well as those with beta-cell destruction that are prone to ketoacidosis for which neither an aetiology nor a pathogenesis is known (idiopathic). Type 2 includes the common major form of diabetes, which results from defect(s) in insulin secretion, almost always with a major contribution from insulin resistance.

Diabetes is a common metabolic disorder which attracts many misconceptions regarding its course and treatment. There is strong convincing evidence to show that good control of blood sugar will reduce the development of the common diabetic complications, including nephropathy, neuropathy, retinopathy and vascular disease. It is now accepted that good diabetic control is achieved by following a healthy balanced diet, taking regular exercise, avoiding too much alcohol and stopping smoking. This advice is common for the entire population and not directed at those people with diabetes.

Challenge 2: Identify why you think it is difficult for Charles to follow a healthy lifestyle

Charles has had a history of eating institutional food, which traditionally has a high fat content and low nutritional value. He is also used to having his food prepared for him and is not experienced in either shopping for or preparing food. He continues to enjoy canteen food and is therefore reluctant to learn how to prepare and cook for himself. He considers what most nutritionists describe as healthy food to be effete.

Charles also believes that he is physically fit, having spent years 'walking the beat' as a policeman and is reluctant to engage in any organised forms of exercise. He believes it to be unnecessary for him. Charles is used to his lifestyle and any suggestions regarding changes to his behaviour tend to make him feel challenged and uncomfortable.

Challenge 3: How can you persuade Charles to review his current behaviour?

The terms *multiprofessional, interdisciplinary* and *multidisciplinary* are often used synonymously. The multiprofessional team consists of a range of different health care professionals and social care professionals who work together for the benefit of the patient. The core team involved with Charles's care may include a diabetic consultant, a diabetic nurse specialist, a dietitian and podiatrists, who would meet to assess and review the provision of care and advice being provided. Others are included as required, for example clinical psychologists, prosthetists, microbiologists and so on. Successful multiprofessional teamwork learning involves the development of shared strategies for clinical and professional interventions. Each member of the team will contribute a specialist understanding of their roles and will develop an understanding of each other's role. They will also contribute team-working skills and positive attitudes, which afford successful interprofessional interaction.

The team involved in the diabetic care of Charles are all actively involved in providing support and reinforcing appropriate behaviours. In order for Charles to achieve his goals, he needs to be provided with information delivered in a way that will enable him to see the personal benefits of changing his behaviours without compromising his lifestyle. His treatment plan should be designed in such a way that offers him small, achievable targets towards the achievement of the overall goal. Positive reinforcements are essential at each stage of the treatment plan and these should be carefully determined and agreed with Charles. All messages should be kept short. When written information is given to Charles, it should be presented in a comprehensible form. Changes to Charles's lifestyle are more likely to occur if they can be integrated into his daily routine.

The podiatrist has an important role to play in contributing to health promotion and health education in podiatry. It is know that systematic and regular foot care and education have been shown to reduce the risk of chronic ulceration and amputation by 50% (Singh *et al.*, 2005).

To improve his health, Charles does not need to give up his visits to the police social club, but simply needs to choose healthier options on the menu, and to moderate his alcohol intake. In addition, Charles would be helped by taking up a hobby which involved an element of physical exercise, such as walking or cycling. Charles may wish to begin by walking at least some of the way to and from his club.

Self-help groups, such as Diabetes UK, offer useful help to people who are newly diagnosed with diabetes. Such groups offer their members support, information, guidance and friendship from other people with diabetes. Increasingly, patients are using recommended web sites from the Internet to gather information about their conditions. The Internet also offers the opportunity to exchange views, information and opinions.

There is also an important issue concerning being prepared for retirement and consideration of life after work. For people who have not prepared adequately, retirement may be a stressful event. Giving up work can be perceived as losing something that is very important. Most employees spend a great deal of time at work, invest effort, energy and enthusiasm, and in return gain satisfaction and a sense of belonging and self-worth. When retirement is not planned, or enforced, feelings of loss may trigger physical and emotional reactions. Employment involves decision-making, interacting with others and a certain amount of physical effort of being at work for designated periods.

People previously in senior positions may suffer from the associated loss of status, and may resent the loss of seniority, which may have taken years to acquire. In all cases, retirement is associated with a loss of income. There may also be feelings of a loss of purpose and structure to the day. Employment involves decision-making, interaction with other employees, the experience of the highs and lows of work life and the physical effort of being at work for designated periods. Employees are often known for their role in the workplace, and thus retirement may result in the loss of social identity.

While many people look forward to retirement, it can also be a source of great stress. Many organisations now offer pre-retirement courses to help prepare their employees to make the transition from work to retirement successful.

Summary of important health psychology

Psychosocial models which try to explain behaviour in general may be helpful when considering an individual patient, but advice should be given in the context of patients' individual circumstances.

It is important for Charles to address the issues of retirement and develop interests and activities that will result in him being able to develop a fulfilled and healthier life.

Implications for podiatric management

It is likely that the minor foot problems Charles exhibits can be managed satisfactorily by an assistant. However, the assistant must be under the supervision and delegation of the podiatrist who has direct responsibility for Charles's management. The assistant must work to an agreed treatment plan with well-identified referral criteria should any deterioration be detected. Careful lines of communication must be maintained between all parties in the multidisciplinary team and Charles's progress must be monitored and screened in accordance with best practice for foot care (Diabetes UK, 2006). In common with all interventions, those who are treating Charles must follow evidence-based practice.

Chapter 8

The psychology of personality, addiction and aggression

The tragedy of machismo is that a man is never quite man enough.

Germaine Greer

The psychology of personality, addiction and aggressive behaviours are discussed in the context of James. The psychological responses to pain are also explored.

James Watt is a 31-year-old runner who has been referred for the first time to the podiatrist. The podiatrist is Jenny, a young and recently qualified graduate (see Chapter 2). James is employed as a sales executive for a local insurance company, which he joined straight from school. He has progressed rapidly through the company and feels that he has been successful as a result of hard work. He questions the need for 'university education' as a key to success, and believes that 'everyone could be successful if they work hard enough'. The major part of James's income is derived from commission. He likes this arrangement: he is ambitious, competitive and approaches his work aggressively. James is generally sociable and enjoys bars, pubs and clubs and has a wide circle of friends and associates from his work. He uses the gym two to three times a week, but his major leisure activity is running. James considers himself to be a competitive runner and is a member of the local harriers. He runs, on average, about 30 miles a week. James believes that running keeps him 'sharp' and gives him an 'edge' in both his social and work life. He enjoys female company but finds it difficult to maintain relationships because of his condescending attitude towards women.

James presents with pain in the anterior aspect of the lower limb, which he describes as 'shin splints'. This condition is considered to be an overuse syndrome.

Factors influencing James's behaviour

James works in an environment that he finds stimulating and satisfying, but which is competitive and financially driven. Being fit is extremely important to him because he believes fitness helps him to work more effectively and he likes the 'buzz' that competitive running provides. His body image is very important to him and he feels confident that he has up-to-date knowledge about how to maintain his physique. He presents with a distinct air of arrogance, and is patronising in his manner.

Important psychological theory

Theories of social perception help to describe how instant assessments of patients occur. Work by Asch (1946) suggests that impressions are drawn from general characteristics and that individuals draw upon their own social constructions of beliefs about people. First impressions can be an important influence, and physical attractiveness has been shown to be a significant factor. The more physically attractive an individual is deemed to be, the more likely they are to be perceived as intelligent, competent and sociable. It is important that podiatrists do not make such judgements.

Personality is considered to be sufficiently stable over time and can be assessed in order to predict behaviour. Many writers have proposed models of personality that have attracted proponents and antagonists in equal measure. Friedman and Rosenman (1974) identify two basic personality types, which they use to describe differences in behaviour. They label individuals as either *Type A* or *Type B*, depending on whether they display certain characteristics and behavioural responses. Type A individuals tend to be competitive, achievement-orientated and impatient, hostile and aggressive and have a sense of urgency about tasks. Conversely, Type B individuals are characterised by non-competitiveness, patience and a placid temperament. Although there has been much research into the relationship between Type A personality and disease, in particular coronary heart disease, there is little corresponding work focusing on the effects of a Type B personality. A further personality type (labelled *Type C*) has been posited (Spiegel, 1991), which is characterised by a habitual tendency to suppress emotions. This tendency has been associated with a number of negative health outcomes. For example, in two longitudinal studies Grosarth-Maticek *et al.* (1982) found emotional suppression to be a significant predictor of cancer in women.

However, there is now wide acceptance of the personality structure proposed by McCrae and Costa (1987). They describe five factors which define an individual's personality. This model has come to be known widely as the Five Factor Theory, or Big Five Model. The five factors are:

- **openness to experience**: the extent to which an individual is willing to try new things
- **conscientiousness**: the extent to which the individual tends to be committed to tasks
- **extroversion**: the extent to which an individual is outgoing
- **agreeableness**: the extent to which the individual gets on well with others
- **neuroticism**: individuals scoring highly tend to feel insecure and to worry.

These may be remembered easily by the use of the mnemonic *OCEAN*. The structure proposed by the Big Five Model has been supported by much statistical evidence.

Personality is believed to influence behaviour profoundly. People who score at the extremes, either high or low, on any of the factors described above are likely to present challenges when attempting to alter their behaviour. This will be the case when Jenny works with James Watt.

Challenge 1: What are the psychological factors that need to be taken into account when planning a treatment regime for James?

Jenny must help James to appreciate the importance of modifying his training regime in order to gain full rehabilitation and enable him to return to competitive running. In order to be able to do this effectively, she will need to understand that running competitively is in part a product of his personality. In addition, running provides James with the opportunity to maintain his appearance, which he values highly.

Runner's high is a recognised state found in long-distance runners. Endorphins are neurotransmitters that are chemically similar to morphine, and are thought to be responsible for elevating mood and reducing pain, particularly after intense periods of exercise such as running. Running has also been associated with feelings of invincibility and superiority (Weston, 1996). The physiological 'high' produced by endorphins in runners is an additional reinforcement of his running behaviour. Research by Aidman and Woollard (2003) indicates that competitive runners show significantly increased withdrawal-like symptoms of depressed mood, reduced vigour and increased tension, anger, fatigue and confusion, within 24 hours of missing a training session.

Negative consequences and contraindications

Compulsive training

Like any activity, exercise can have its downside. Overuse of any coping strategy can create additional problems. For some, physical activity can be escape from taking responsibility for one's actions. By indulging themselves in their activity, individuals avoid troubling life situations that are difficult to resolve. Similarly, although most can benefit from increased levels of self-esteem, this is different from the unhealthy narcissistic tendencies others derive from physical training.

Aggressive tendencies

Although physical activity can be a useful catharsis for aggression, aggressive sporting activities can act to condition one to become more aggressive. If one learns to be successful by acting overly aggressively, it is not a far stretch to see how some may use this aggression to get what they want in other areas of life.

Addiction

Those who exercise on a daily basis often describe being addicted to their activity. Although considered to be a positive addiction to some, the withdrawal effects of not being able to exercise can create problems. Whether caused by changes in catecholamine levels (not getting their daily fix of endorphins) or some other mechanism, individuals should be aware of possible increases in hostility, anxiety, irritability and depression associated with not working out.

It is necessary, therefore, to identify an alternative means of meeting these needs on a temporary basis while James stops running in order for resolution of his condition to take place. Although the initial need for rest is of paramount importance, replacement activities must also be considered, discussed and negotiated.

James's personality is such that he is likely to demand simple answers to solve his problem, thereby enabling him to carry on his fitness regime. Jenny will be helped in this task by an understanding of personality theory and how personality may influence health-related behaviour. Jenny's approach should thus be a combination of empathy and assertiveness.

Jenny's task is complicated further by the interaction of James's personality and the pain he experiences. Pain is a common experience and is inseparable from everyday life. Physiologically, pain can be considered as an unpleasant sensory and emotional experience associated with actual or potential tissue damage. The physiological process of pain is described extensively in appropriate texts and is not the focus of this book. Understanding psychological responses to pain is very important for podiatrists. The way in which an individual responds to pain will vary according to certain factors, which are outlined below.

Factors affecting pain perception

The following factors will all impact on the experience and expression of pain:

- social and cultural background
- previous experiences of pain
- the responses of significant others to pain
- emotional effects
- the perceived intensity of the pain
- the ability to communicate and describe the pain
- permission to express pain in the culture
- the efficacy of pain-relieving drugs.

Interprofessional communication

It is important to establish James's source of referral and his treatment history. If he has sought the advice of several other professionals prior to being referred to the podiatrist, it will be important for Jenny to obtain this information early on and determine the nature of the advice he has been given. If the advice Jenny provides is congruent with advice James has been given earlier, then he is more likely to follow it.

Jenny's communication style needs to be confident, knowledgeable and sensitive to James's needs. She should be aware of, and understand, the factors that make running so important to him. It is also necessary for James to listen actively to the advice Jenny gives in order that an agreed treatment plan can be devised.

Challenge 2: Identify the potential problems you may encounter with James and how you would overcome them

Addictive behaviours

Addiction is a term that is often used somewhat loosely, and some authors have pointed out that it is not only substances such as alcohol, nicotine and opiates that have addictive properties. Many of the features of such substances can also be seen in certain behaviours, notably in the case of athletic and sporting endeavours. In a slightly whimsical overview of the debate, Miller and Marlatt (1977) describe a screening test for an addictive state they describe as 'Skiism'. They observe that skiing is 'a winter sport/addictive behaviour of major proportions', and note that its victims persist with their addiction 'in spite of the ever-increasing cost of their habit, and seemingly oblivious to the steady stream of ambulances that carry off the casualties of intemperance and over-exposure'. Miller and Marlatt propose a psychological self-assessment scale which suggests that positive responses to such questions as 'Has skiing ever separated you from your family?' and 'Do you find that it takes progressively stiffer slopes to satisfy you?' to indicate a condition which Stepney (1981) describes as 'the features of escapism, development of tolerance, and personal and social dislocation which characterize a full-blown dependence disorder'. Symptoms of exercise addiction can also include non-compliance, aggression and the need to continually seek advice from different health care professionals.

Runners frequently become addicted to running and continue to run even when it is detrimental to their health (Chapman and De Castro, 1990). Running addiction can now be measured using the Running Addiction Scale (RAS). This scale is a validated research tool that is used to investigate the psychological correlates of running addiction. The RAS consists of a symptom checklist, details of the individual's running habits and the degree of their addiction (Chapman and De Castro, 1990).

Viewed from this perspective, the notion of a jogging addiction seems less absurd than a first glance may suggest. James exhibits many features of addictive behaviour, and it is important that Jenny give them adequate consideration when agreeing the treatment plan.

Aggression

Aggression may manifest itself in many forms, the nature of which may be mediated by factors such gender, age and culture. Aggression may be considered as behaviour or speech intended to harm someone else, to obtain material goods or as a reaction to another person's aggressive behaviour.

Research indicates that men have a tendency to be more aggressive than women, largely because of their different characteristic levels of the hormone testosterone. However, Bjorkqvist et al. (1992) studied physical, verbal and indirect aggression (such as gossiping and writing unkind notes) in adolescent males and females. They found that boys displayed higher levels of physical aggression but that girls showed significantly higher levels of indirect aggression. Boys and girls showed no difference in their levels of verbal aggression.

One of the most influential approaches to understanding aggression is Social Learning Theory, first proposed by Bandura (1973). This theory suggests that aggressive behaviour is the product of *observational learning*, or copying the behaviour of others. Bandura's theory is limited in that it does not take into account factors such as a person's affective state, their personality or their interpretation of the situation. A subsequent theory of aggression has been proposed by proponents of Social Constructionism. Social constructionists, such as Gergen (1997), believe that people impose subjective interpretations, or constructions, on the environment surrounding them. When applied to aggression, Social Constructionism is based on the following assumptions:

- Aggressive behaviour is a form of social behaviour and is not simply an expression of anger.
- Our interpretation or construction of someone else's behaviour as aggressive or non-aggressive depends on our beliefs and knowledge.
- Our decision on whether to behave aggressively or non-aggressively depends on how we interpret the other person's behaviour to us.

(Gergen, 1997)

The value of this approach is that it takes into consideration the effect of attitudes and beliefs and the need to distinguish between what actually happens in a social situation and what is perceived to happen. Conversely, a criticism that could be applied is that social constructionist approaches may exaggerate the differences between different individuals' constructions of what has occurred.

All health care practitioners have an important role to play in helping to achieve concordance with negotiated treatment plans. Providing patients with clear, honest explanations and advice, while being sensitive to their individual needs, promotes concordance (Pitts, 1991). Other strategies include the keeping of diaries, graduating the complexity of the prescribed regimen, marrying the requirements of the regimen to daily activities and finding alternatives to the behaviour which the patient finds difficult to change. For example, James could use weights or swim in order to maintain his fitness during this necessary period of rest.

Summary of important health psychology

The important psychological issues in this case study surround the manifestations of James's personality on his behaviour. James obtains satisfaction from the challenges that he has introduced to his life, which include working on a commission basis and the competitive nature of his relaxation activities. An understanding of his nature and motivations will enable Jenny to build a rehabilitation programme with which James is likely to be concordant. In addition, she must understand and acknowledge that patients will interpret pain differently and respond to it in individual ways.

Implications for podiatric management

The diagnosis of overuse syndrome initially would indicate that rest is of optimum importance. Nevertheless, it is imperative to make a full assessment of James's foot and lower-limb functions. Many podiatrists have extended scope skills in sports medicine and musculoskeletal management and are part of a multidisciplinary team. Where this is not the case, it may well be wise for the podiatrist to refer to experts. The use of video analysis and of other forms of movement analysis may be able to identify anomalies in James's gait which would benefit from intervention. As previously indicated, such work is performed by a specialist podiatrist. Jenny must decide, therefore, whether she has the ability to manage James herself or should refer him. Such judgements require good reflective and clinical-reasoning skills, both of which Jenny possesses.

Chapter 9

Communication through an interpreter

*Shallow understanding from people of good will is more
frustrating than absolute misunderstanding from people
of ill will.*

Martin Luther King, Jr.

Sheetal Joshi is a patient who has suffered a stroke and who does not
speak English. Communication with her is via a family member acting as
interpreter. This chapter explores the issues arising from this situation.

Sheetal is a 70-year-old Asian lady, originally from the Indian subconti-
nent. She is dressed in a traditional style of clothing, which covers her head,
arms and legs. Sheetal is a small, slightly overweight, grey-haired lady who
had a stroke about a year ago which affected the right side of her body. Her
arm is in a flexed position, her gait is affected and she has to walk with the
aid of a walking stick.

Sheetal lives with her extended family in a predominantly Asian community in London. She is accompanied by her daughter-in-law, Hetal, who
speaks good English and, since Sheetal was widowed, acts as her interpreter.
Sheetal both communicates through Hetal and consults her when asked
questions. She does not maintain eye contact with anyone other than her
daughter-in-law, and looks to her for confirmation that her responses are
'correct'. Sheetal believes that her stroke and resultant disability are 'God's
way of testing her faith'.

Hetal reports that since having had her stroke her mother-in-law has
become depressed, and that she is reluctant to go out of the house. Sheetal
is afraid of falling and feels that if she were to have an accident she would no
be able to make herself understood in order to get help. Hetal also reports

that her mother-in-law feels frustrated by her lack of improvement over the last few months.

Sheetal has been referred to you for an assessment of her foot health and rehabilitation options. She has been referred to the rehabilitation team in which you are working. Her doctor is concerned about her vascular status, and the care of her feet. He has referred her for advice and treatment, which may include orthotic management.

Factors influencing Sheetal's behaviour

Asian people living in the United Kingdom have been found to have high rates of stroke, which are attributed to high dietary salt and sugar intake (Enas *et al.*, 1996, 1997). Stroke is the leading form of cardiovascular disease in Asian populations (Enas *et al.*, 1997).

A stroke is a disruption in the blood supply to the brain. It is frequently referred to as a *cerebrovascular accident*, or CVA for short. It is also discussed in terms of *left CVA* or *right CVA*, referring to the left or right hemisphere of the brain. If the disruption is temporary and blood flow is restored without any residual or remaining difficulty, then the episode is known as a *transient ischaemic attack* (TIA). If the blood supply to the brain is not restored, permanent damage to the affected brain tissue will ensue, which leads to the muscular dysfunctions and deformities associated with stroke.

Asian people living in the United Kingdom are known to use health services less often and suffer more from premature death, disease and disabilities than do people born in the United Kingdom. Many also face social, economic and cultural barriers to maintaining good health. Because ethnic minority groups in the United Kingdom are very diverse, women's access to health care, their health behaviours and their health status can vary widely. Depression is a commonly reported psychological outcome of stroke.

Sheetal is a devout Muslim and therefore would find exposing any part of her body to a male podiatrist unacceptable; Sheetal would be less likely to feel this way with a female podiatrist. This is the first time you have met Sheetal and her daughter-in-law. The letter of referral that you have received provides limited information and only a sketchy medical history.

It is important for the podiatrist to have an understanding of the relevant cultural issues in order to be able to provide Sheetal with appropriate podiatric care and advice; communication is therefore key. Anthropological studies have demonstrated that when two people who do not share the same cultural framework communicate with each other there is a higher probability of misunderstanding occurring. Culture, therefore, contextualises what is said. In many cultures, the provision of consent does not always mean agreement. It can be given to avoid upsetting the other person. This is contrary to the Western custom of directly asking questions. Communication is also a process of exchange. In some cultures, an intimate conversation between a therapist and their patient is seen to be strange. It may be more common to talk in the presence of family or friends who not only listen but also give their opinion. In addition, talking about personal matters in a first interview may be disturbing and so an informal pre-meeting may be preferred, during which refreshments can be offered and where the two parties can get to know each other. Non-verbal communication may also be different. In Western cultures, it is common for participants to look at each other and maintain eye contact; however, in some non-Western cultures, people look away as a sign of respect.

Important psychosocial factors

Sheetal's religious and cultural background would make her very unwilling to expose any part of her body to a male podiatrist. She may ask if there is a female podiatrist available, but this should be anticipated and provided without the need for her to make such a request. Sheetal's attitudes towards her health will be closely interwoven with her religious beliefs.

South Asians living in the United Kingdom (Indians, Bangladeshis, Pakistanis and Sri Lankans) have a higher premature death rate from coronary heart disease than average. The rate is 46% higher for men and 51% higher for women.

The difference in the death rates between South Asians and the rest of the British population is increasing as the mortality rate in Asian people is not falling as fast as it is in the rest of the population. From 1971 to 1991, the mortality rate for 20- to 69-year-olds for the whole population fell by 29% for men and 17% for women. In South Asian people, it fell by 20% for men and 7% for women. South Asian people also have a mortality rate from stroke which is 55% higher than average for men and 41% higher for women.

The association between depression and stroke is well established in terms of the negative impact of a stroke on an individual's rehabilitation, family relationships, and their subsequent quality of life. The early diagnosis and treatment of depression can shorten the rehabilitation period, and lead to a more rapid recovery and resumption of routine daily activities.

Conducting an interview through an interpreter will require more time than would a similar interaction with an English-speaking patient. This should be borne in mind when allocating appointment times. Some of the finer points of the conversation may be lost in interpretation. Moreover, people from different cultures may use non-verbal signals in ways that may be unfamiliar or open to misinterpretation. Interpreters have the responsibility of passing on complex information or material that is personal or sensitive in nature, and about which the patient may have to make decisions.

The use of an interpreter may result in the patient feeling embarrassed or intimidated, particularly if the interpreter is from a higher social class, or as in Sheetal's case a family member. If the interpreter is from the same community as the patient, there might be anxieties concerning the disclosure of intimate family matters, and associated issues of confidentiality (Karseras and Hopkins, 1987). In addition, Hetal may be embarrassed by her mother-in-law's inability to speak English and her possible lack of understanding about her condition and may wish to compensate by implying understanding on Sheetal's part that, in reality, does not exist.

Traditionally, in South Asian families, on marriage the bride lives with her new husband and her in-laws, and regards her mother-in-law as a mentor who will provide guidance and advice. Mothers and wives have clearly defined roles within the family unit. However, during her visit to the clinic, these roles are reversed. Sheetal is completely dependent upon Hetal's ability to speak English and may thus feel powerless. By contrast, Hetal may feel apprehensive about accepting this atypical role with the responsibility of ensuring satisfactory provision of her mother-in-law's health care.

Challenge 1: How can you feel confident that the information and advice you offer is understood and that the patient's needs are being understood?

The tripartite nature of the consultation may lead to Hetal translating verbatim, interpreting the messages and responses or a mixture of all of these. This may lead to inaccuracies in the understandings between Sheetal and the podiatrist, which may result in inappropriate treatment and advice.

There is no direct communication between the podiatrist and Sheetal; all communication occurs through Hetal (Figure 9.1). In the process of interpretation, many subtleties of conversation may be lost. The relative emphasis placed on different components in the exchange, for example history-taking, severity and duration of symptoms (from Sheetal via Hetal to the podiatrist) and information, advice and education (from the podiatrist to Sheetal via Hetal) may be altered. This may result in a compromised outcome for both patient and podiatrist. A useful technique that may be helpful in this situation is to invite the interpreter to paraphrase your original message from time to time during the consultation.

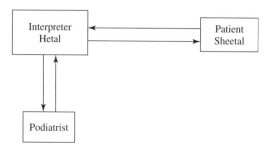

Figure 9.1 Communication and the interpreter

Habermas (1989) has analysed communication techniques in order to identify communication difficulties. He defines four key points to help interpret communication difficulties. These include:

- lack of intelligibility
- disagreement about a problem
- unacceptable behaviour
- distrust and lack of sincerity in the relationship.

These difficulties help to explain how lack of clarity or a misunderstanding of an opinion can be interpreted as a disagreement, and how a behaviour may be perceived as unacceptable, which can result in a misunderstanding. All of these are more likely and more probable in cross-cultural interactions, given that language, behaviour, codes and meaning are all different.

Moreover, cultural differences, emotional tensions and lack of language are further complicated by working with an interpreter. Interpreters are necessary where there are language barriers to help ease communication as well as translate cultural concepts and ways of understanding things. An interpreter will ideally have an understanding of:

- the beliefs, norms and values of the culture
- the relationship of the person to authority
- the relationship between the individual and the family
- a culture's understanding of and approach to death and dying
- the hierarchy and roles within the social structure, defined positions, expected conduct and punishable behaviours for people
- the importance of symbols and rituals.

Challenge 2: Consider the central role of religious belief in people's lives

Many studies have demonstrated the positive effects of religiosity on a wide range of health outcomes, for example reductions in coronary heart disease (Koenig, 1998; Koenig *et al.*, 1998), hypertension and cancer (Levin, 1994).

Positive and negative religious coping

One study suggested that faith-based, positive religious resources could help patients recover from cardiac surgery (American Psychological Association, 2006). Results indicate that enhanced hope and perceived social support can protect psychological well-being during stressful procedures and experiences, whereas having negative religious thoughts and struggles may hinder recovery.

In the study, acts of positive religious coping were defined as religious forgiveness, seeking spiritual support, collaborative religious coping or fellowship with others who share the same beliefs, spiritual connection, religious purification and thoughts of religious benevolence. Negative coping styles included spiritual discontent, thoughts of punishing God, insecurity, demonic thoughts, interpersonal religious discontent, religious doubt and discontented spiritual relations.

Positive religious coping styles had positive effects on both hope and social support, whereas negative styles were inversely related to social support. Perceived social support and hope contributed to less depression and anxiety for postoperative patients who used positive religious coping styles. Negative, but not positive, religious coping styles were also directly related to postoperative distress. Religiousness contributed only to positive, and not to negative, religious coping styles, but there was no direct effect of religiousness on social support, hope or postoperative distress.

Besides being related to poor postoperative recovery, the negative effect of religious doubts was also manifest through hopelessness and lower levels of perceived social support before stressful experiences such as cardiac surgery. There is also a suggestion that religious struggles, linked to poor mental health, predicted mortality (Pargament *et al.*, 2001).

Early attention to such impacts can lead to an appropriate intervention, and as a result long-term harm may be prevented. Clarifying the psychosocial mechanisms of potential protective and harmful faith influences will enable health and mental health professionals to work collaboratively in order to enhance disease management and health promotion.

It is therefore important to understand the centrality of religion or spirituality in many people's lives as something other than a potential barrier to treatment. The relationship of spirituality to health is explored in greater depth in Chapter 22.

Summary of important health psychology

The podiatrist will require sensitivity and patience in order to meet Sheetal's needs. Her inability to speak English and the residual effects of her recent stroke will make communication difficult. In addition, cultural and religious understanding is essential to Sheetal's successful rehabilitation. The podiatrist will also have to acknowledge that she is part of a multidisciplinary team. Multidisciplinary team-working requires mutual understanding between professions. Good communication, positive attitudes and a common goal are also necessary for a successful outcome.

Implications for podiatric management

Sheetal is consulting a multidisciplinary rehabilitation team. In cases such as hers, the consequences of stroke is often dropped foot and accompanying neuromuscular and vascular complications. Sheetal's assessment is likely to identify the need for close cooperation with the shoemaker, and the provision of an ankle foot orthosis. In some cases, the consequences of stroke are such that the use of a calliper may be required in order to reduce the effects of drop foot. The deformities resulting from the neuromuscular effects may result in areas of high pressure, commonly over the lateral border of the foot with resultant callus and corn formation. Treatment planning must include decisions regarding the treatment of skin lesions, the provision of palliative foot care and, importantly, orthotics which may improve mobility. In addition, regular screening and evaluation of vascular status and skin patency must be undertaken. All of these must be achieved within the supportive context of the multidisciplinary team and provide Sheetal with confidence that her ambitions for rehabilitation are acknowledged and can be met.

Chapter 10

The psychological effects of bereavement

If two people love each other there can be no happy end to it.

Ernest Hemingway

Enid Hilton has recently experienced the unexpected death of her husband. The psychological effects of dying and death are explored in this chapter.

Enid is a lady who has moved from the Midlands to the south coast to retire with her husband. She has been living in the town with her husband in a small flat for 10 years. She is a smart, slender lady who always seems to wear a hat and coat and low-heeled, black patent leather court shoes. She has a slightly nervous disposition and was always accompanied by her husband to her podiatry appointments. Her husband was always reported as being her 'rock' and undertook all the financial responsibilities of their married life.

Since Enid's last appointment, her husband suffered a short illness and died unexpectedly. As a result of this, her nervousness has been exacerbated and she is displaying signs of stress. Since Enid's last appointment, there has been a change in the local Trust's policy, and she is no longer eligible for state-funded treatment. This situation has to be explained to her at her final appointment with the podiatrist.

Podiatric presentation

Enid has cold, thin, bony feet, with bunions, lesser-toe deformity, corns and calluses. She has an uneventful medical history.

Factors influencing Enid's behaviour

Enid has just experienced the death of a loved one. Both the death and the events leading up to it might have had a range of physical and psychological effects, and for some these can be devastating.

Enid is in a state of confusion and feels extremely vulnerable at the loss of her long-time partner and friend. As a result of this, she is demonstrating some of the signs of stress, reporting that she frequently cries and blames herself for her husband's death. She has feelings of being disempowered and no longer in control of her life.

Bereavement forces the bereaved person to accommodate significant changes that can have a major impact on their social identity. In order for the podiatrist to help Enid and to communicate with her effectively, it is important to have an understanding of the psychological impact of death and dying and the stages associated with the bereavement process.

The processes of dying and death

Older people may be expected to be more accepting of death than younger people as they are more likely to have considered the consequences, and even prepared for the event. However, when the process of dying occurs unexpectedly, the impact may be more profound.

The anticipated loss of a partner can give rise to feelings of vulnerability, which stem from fear and anger. Fear originates typically as a reaction to not being able to cope alone and the prospect of an unknown future. Conversely, anger can provide patients with a mechanism to cope with their grief, but it can also be destructive, especially when the aggression is directed towards family members or health care professionals. Anger is an understandable reaction and arises from feelings of intense personal frustration and the blocking of personal goals (Berkowitz, 1993). However, Weiner (1986) points out that anger and aggression often stem from a sense of injustice and a belief that others are to blame. This is a common reaction and appears to reflect a fundamental human need to find an explanation for untoward events. Kübler-Ross (1969), in a seminal work based on studies of studying dying patients, challenges the taboo of discussing dying. From this work, she has helped to identify her patients' needs.

The process through which a bereaved person moves is extensively described by Parkes (1986) and Kübler-Ross (1969).

Kübler-Ross describes five stages of dying (Box 10.1).

Box 10.1 Kübler-Ross's five stages of dying

Stage	Behavioural response
Denial	This is often the first reaction on receiving the news that life is limited.
Anger	The patient may try to blame others, including health care professionals.
Bargaining	The patient may promise to change their behaviour, to be good or compliant or to give up bad habits in return for being able to live longer.
Depression	If death is inevitable, the patient may become depressed and withdrawn and may refuse treatment. They may be anticipating their own death and mourning.
Acceptance	This is the final stage, where the patient is resigned and may wish to say farewell.

Source: Adapted from Kübler-Ross, 1969.

These stages are not chronological and not all of the stages are experienced by all people.

Bereavement is the term for the loss of a loved one and is followed by a response that is known as the *grief reaction*. Parkes (1986) studied widows in the first year of their bereavement, which led him to break down the grieving process into four stages (Box 10.2).

Box 10.2 Parkes' stages of grief reaction

Stage	Behavioural response
Denial	This stage is typified by feelings of numbness and a lack of reality. The bereaved may cry a lot, feel embarrassed and feel that crying is an inappropriate behaviour. Mourning is a cultural expression of grief and so will vary between different cultures.
Yearning	The bereaved may want to hold onto personal items from the dead person, such as clothing, letters or mementos.
Despair	Feelings of despair may be intense and result in depression. In some cases, the spouse may feel life is not worth living without their partner.
Recovery	This is the gradual acceptance of the bereaved state although some report never being able to get over it completely.

Source: Adapted from Alder, 1999.

As with the process of dying, the stages are not fixed but are evident. Events and anniversaries are key times for the bereaved and may rekindle the grieving process. The grief reaction includes emotions of fear, anger, guilt and sadness.

Parkes (1986) argues that fear is caused by a sense of vulnerability and may result in the bereaved person avoiding the stressor that is causing the fear. Anger is caused by a sense of frustration and a belief that others are to blame, and may result in the bereaved person wanting to assign blame. Guilt is caused by a belief that the bereaved person may have failed the person who has died. The bereaved person's reaction is to blame themselves. Intense sadness and feelings of emptiness are caused by the severance of attachment and the loss of an important part of self. Although such models can oversimplify the process and experience of bereavement, they are useful to help understand the emotional stages that patients may experience.

Worden (1991) describes the mechanisms of grief and the procedure for helping patients accomplish the 'tasks of mourning' to facilitate moving through the process. However, Ramsay and de Groot (1977) argue that the processes involved in coming to terms with loss may not be predictable in the staged way that theorists suggest. They propose that there are nine components of grief which may occur in different ways. These include:

- shock or numbness
- disorganisation or an inability to plan
- denial (expecting the spouse to return home)
- depression
- guilt at having neglected the spouse or for treating them badly
- anxiety about the future
- aggression (towards doctors or family)
- resolution or acceptance of the situation
- reintegration into life.

Counsellors working with bereaved people also report that it is common-place for the bereaved to see and/or hear the person who has died with remarkable clarity.

The final stage of grief is that of recovery, although Stroebe et al. (1993) suggest that complete recovery is often impossible. They propose that when 'there has been strong attachment to the lost one, involvement is likely to continue, even for a lifetime'.

Stroebe (2001) suggests that the loss of a partner affects the survivor's social functioning in four main ways, involving, as it does, a loss of:

- social and emotional support
- social validation of their personal judgements

- material and task support (in most marriages, there is role differentiation; after bereavement, the survivor has to take on all roles)
- social protection.

Difficulties in adjustment to being bereaved may manifest themselves in other ways. It is well established that a sharp increase in consultations with general practitioners occurs following the death of a partner. There is also an increase in reported physical symptomatology among widowed people, accompanied by a 40% increase in mortality rate in the six months following a spouse's death (Prigerson *et al.*, 1997). Widowed people report behavioural problems with their children, which Silverman and Worden (1993) ascribe these to poor adjustment strategies adopted by the surviving parent. Although there are several explanations for such findings, including reduction in immunocompetence, there are many who report that such symptoms and behaviours occur as a result of a 'broken heart'.

Challenge 1: Explain to Enid the reasons why her state-funded treatment is being removed. Consider the effects this will have on her treatment in the future

Enid no longer qualifies for state-funded treatment. It is necessary for you to discharge her from your care. It is inevitable that the practitioner employed in the state sector is likely to be subject to changes in funding arrangements as a result of political change. This will change the nature of the service that the podiatrist is able to provide; in real terms, this will mean a reduction in the availability of care. The responsibility for implementing these policies, and explaining the outcomes to patients, falls to the practitioner.

Consider how you would inform Enid that she must be discharged.

- Consider the impact of bereavement and the stages that individuals go through following bereavement.
- Consider the boundaries between giving podiatric advice, general health advice and counselling.
- Consider how the involvement of others in the health, social work and voluntary sector teams may have a role in the care of bereaved people.
- Consider the needs of the podiatrist in this situation.

Challenge 2: What factors will affect Enid as a result of her loss of contact with the podiatrist?

Enid has found her contact with you to be very supportive since her recent bereavement. Because of the new policy, this contact will be terminated abruptly. What alternatives for support can be offered? What are the important psychological factors to be considered in Enid's case?

To be empowered is to have a good sense of identity and to feel that one has control over things that really matter. It also involves caring about others and feelings of belonging and of being accepted. Empowerment includes feeling being valued and being able to make a real contribution. Conversely, to feel disempowered is to feel insignificant, with a sense that life has little meaning, and to have little control over things that really matter. People with a low sense of empowerment may feel socially excluded and like an outsider in the society in which they live.

Stress can be said to be the result of a stressor such as an adverse life event which results in a response which has physical, emotional and behavioural components. Enid is currently experiencing high levels of stress. This will make her more vulnerable to the onset of illness. There is evidence that the immune system is compromised after prolonged periods of severe stress, and clearly Enid is very vulnerable. Moreover, should she become ill, she would have greatly reduced resources to deal with her illness.

Early models of stress proposed by Seyle (1950) and Lazarus (1966) only considered physiological responses to stressors but did not examine the nature of stressors themselves. Cox (1978) later developed a transactional model of stress, in which he suggests that stress depends on the interaction between an individual and their environment. Cox proposes that the stress an individual experiences is the product of both the nature of the stressor and the individual's perception of their ability to cope with it. Perceived stress is therefore a highly subjective experience, and different people will react differently to similar stressors. This work has been echoed by Steptoe (1997), who proposes that stress 'responses are said to arise when demands exceed personal and social resources that the individual is able to mobilise'.

Coping resources and an individual's vulnerability (McEwan and Stellar, 1993) are considered to be central to the relationship between stress and health. Predisposing biological and psychosocial factors and vulnerability play a dual role in the mechanism by which stress influences health. Physiological, behavioural and psychological processes may directly influence health in specific ways. For example, stress has measurable effects on the autonomic nervous system. Neuroendocrine mediators influence immune, gastrointestinal, neuromuscular and cardiovascular systems (McEwan, 1998). Acute activation of these systems is known to precipitate short-term adaptive physiological changes as well as a whole range of somatic symptoms, which can manifest as an increased heart rate, increased perspiration and gastrointestinal motility. These symptoms may then be interpreted as being indicative of illness.

Although physiological activation has short-term adaptive benefits, any chronic activation of these systems is believed to enhance vulnerability to cardiovascular, metabolic, immune-related and other diseases (Chrousos and Gold, 1992). In addition, such chronic activation results in changes in the central nervous system and brain (Sapolsky, 1996). Behavioural responses such as changes in eating, sleeping, consumption of alcohol and other substances can increase the risk of illness and disease. Psychological symptoms include altered self-perception and heightened awareness of body sensations. These sensations normally go unrecognised but may be interpreted as indicators of illness (Pennebaker, 1982).

The links between stress and ill health have been questioned by some authors. In particular, it has been pointed out that many of the studies which demonstrate such a link have been retrospective in nature. This means that, whilst a clear association can be demonstrated to exist between stress and illness, data concerning stress and illness are gathered at the same time. Thus, while stress and illness co-occur, it is difficult to demonstrate that stress causes illness rather than the illness resulting in stress. In prospective studies, measures of stress are taken before illness occurs and are compared with illness at a later date. If a relationship is demonstrated in this way, it would seem reasonable (although not certain) to conclude that stress is likely to cause illness rather than vice versa.

Such criticisms, however, may represent a simplistic approach in which stressful events are deemed to be the sole cause of disease, rather than contributory factors which may alter *susceptibility* to disease (Dowrenwend *et al.*, 1982; Walker and Katon, 1990).

Summary of important health psychology

An understanding of the process of dying, death and bereavement is fundamental for the podiatrist to be able to respond to Enid's needs. Reactions to actual or anticipated loss are complex and mediated by individual differences. Staged models are useful tools which help to explain the experiences of bereaved people. However, it is also important to recognise that not all such people will respond in the manner proposed by such models. Patients will draw on their resources to cope with the trauma of bereavement. Such resources may include social support, the individual's characteristics, personality traits and habitual methods of dealing with stressful events.

The time taken for an individual to recover from bereavement varies widely and for most people the process is never truly complete. However, if acute grief persists for longer than 18 months to two years, this may be an indication that some form of help may be valuable. It is important for the podiatrist to recognise when such intervention is necessary so that an appropriate referral can be made.

Implications for podiatric management

Enid does not present the podiatrist with a challenging podiatric presentation. However, it is likely that she will still want to have treatment. It is the responsibility of the podiatrist in the state-funded service to enable the efficient and effective transfer from state-provided services to either the independent or voluntary sector for foot health care. Enid must be equipped with such advice regarding the care of her feet, footwear and the prevention and consequences of the cold on her feet prior to discharge. It must also be made clear how, should her condition change or deteriorate or should she develop a systemic disorder, that Enid can access the state service once again.

Enid may perceive being discharged from the service as a further loss, and the podiatrist needs to be sensitive to this possibility. During the discharge interview, broader aspects of Enid's needs may be discussed and those agencies which are available to help Enid can be identified. The podiatrist should also have available lists of appropriate referents and agencies and suitably qualified podiatrists in independent practice. In addition, the podiatrist should offer to make formal introductions and provide referral letters.

Chapter 11

The relationship between socio-economic status and health

Equality is the public recognition, effectively expressed in institutions and manners, of the principle that an equal degree of attention is due to the needs of all human beings.

Simone Weil

The relationship between socio-economic status and health is investigated using the character of Bill Canning.

Bill is a 60-year-old school caretaker who is married and has four grown-up children, all of whom have moved away from home. He lives in a small, two-bedroom ex-council house, which he has just completed buying. He works on a part-time basis at the local infant school, where he has been employed for 10 years. The school has only a small number of children, is privately funded and well maintained. Bill is shown little respect by the teaching staff, and the head teacher is particularly patronising towards him. However, the children love him and on the whole he enjoys his work.

Bill is an affable person and likes to socialise with his friends in the local pub. He is partial to 'a pint or two', especially on darts nights. Bill is a smoker who would not consider trying to give up smoking, nor his preference for 'fast food', which has led to him becoming clinically obese. He believes that 'we all have to die from something' and carries this fatalistic view into his everyday life.

Bill is referred to the podiatrist with painful highly arched feet.

Factors influencing Bill's behaviour

Bill's situation presents him with a dilemma. The lifestyle and behaviour that he adopts is different from those who employ and work with him. There are times when he is made to feel uncomfortable as a result of this difference. There are thus three important issues to be considered in Bill's situation. First, the school is funded solely by fee-paying parents. As a result, paying for education and health care is viewed as a matter of individual choice, rather than state-funded education and health care being seen as the foundation of a just society. Moreover, there is strong support for the notion that paying for such services will result in them being better.

Second, Bill is poorly paid in relation to the teaching staff and parents. He does not have the resources to exercise such 'choice'. Finally, Bill believes strongly that he has paid for his health care through taxation, and that having to pay for such services is an abdication of responsibility by the state.

Important psychological theory

Socio-economic status is a term used to describe a person's position in society, and is usually expressed in terms of income, education and occupation. It could also be represented by net worth, ownership of assets such as a home, car or other material possessions. By any such classification, Bill belongs to a lower socio-economic group than do his work colleagues and the children's parents.

The British population is generally more affluent than ever before. However, there is still little social mobility between the social classes. The most commonly used classification of socio-economic status is that proposed by the Registrar General's Classification of Occupations. This framework classifies people according to their employment:

- **Class I**: higher professional (e.g. medicine, law, architecture)
- **Class II**: lower professional (e.g. nursing, podiatry, physiotherapy, management)
- **Class IIIN**: skilled non-manual (e.g. secretarial workers, administrators)
- **Class IIIM**: skilled manual (e.g. plumbers, electricians, mechanics)
- **Class IV**: semi-skilled (e.g. postal workers, bus drivers, shop assistants)
- **Class V**: unskilled (e.g. porters, refuse collectors).

Minor modifications have been made to this scale from time to time, but it remains the method of classification used in the majority of British studies published in the last two decades.

It is important to note that this classification has a number of limitations. For example, in studies of families or couples the social class of the unit is generally defined by the occupation of the male partner. Second, some occupations in lower social groups are actually better paid than some found in higher groups.

There is much evidence which demonstrates that health status is unequal across different groups in British society (Townsend and Davidson, 1982). Research suggests that health is related to geographical location, gender, age and socio-economic status. Since the 1980s, it has been recognised that poorer people have poorer health than those who are better off. Attention has been paid to this effect since the publication of the *Black Report* in England in 1980 (Townsend and Davidson, 1982). Subsequent studies have demonstrated that this disparity in health status remains, even when behavioural differences such as smoking, diet and physical activity are controlled. It is clear that there is a direct relationship between social deprivation and poorer health status (Beale, 2001).

Other authors have examined the relationship between income and morbidity, both before and after controlling for other socio-economic variables (Ecob and Davey Smith, 1999). This study used data taken from the Health and Lifestyle National Survey of adults aged 18, which was conducted in 1984/5. It resulted in 9003 interviews being performed which included questions concerning the material circumstances of the respondents. The results suggest that health is linearly related to income: *as income increases so health improves.* A further dimension to this is the size and quality of people's housing. Dunn and Hayes (2000) investigated two independent neighbourhoods in Vancouver. They found that both quality of housing and available living area per head of occupant were positively associated not only with socio-economic status but also with health status. Dunn and Hayes (2000) suggest that the circumstances of an individual's housing play an important role in determining their social status and social identity.

Other studies exist which demonstrate that a fear of illness and injury are much more common in patients from lower socio-economic classes (Noyes *et al.*, 2000). Moreover, there is evidence to suggest that people in such circumstances utilise health care services in a different way from those in higher socio-economic groups. People of lower socio-economic status receive less health care from the British National Health Service than do those from higher socio-economic classes (Le Grand, 1993).

The NHS was originally set up to provide treatment free at the point of delivery irrespective of the patient's ability to pay. Although this ethic is still ostensibly maintained, there are occasions where either particular forms of health care fall outside the remit of the NHS or patients may opt to use private health care. This has resulted in a situation which is quite different from the original concept of the NHS.

The relationship between ability to pay for health care and the willingness to pay for it is complex and has been explored in only a few studies

(Russell, 1996; Donaldson, 1999). However, this may become increasingly contentious as the nature of NHS provision changes in line with political thought.

The most common means of measuring inequalities in health status is known as the Standardised Mortality Ratio (or SMR). This is calculated as follows:

$$\frac{\text{The observed death rate in a given population}}{\text{The expected death rate in that population}} \times 100$$

Thus, a population which displays more illness than would be expected has an SMR which is greater than 100, and a population which displays less illness than would be expected has an SMR of less than 100. In all cases, the death rate may be controlled for the age distribution of the population. Over 20 years, the *Black Report* first demonstrated the SMR in the highest social class to be 77 for men and 82 for women, while the SMR in the poorest section of the population was 137 for men and 135 for women. It is known that this discrepancy has widened alarmingly since the publication of the *Black Report*.

Challenge 1: Refer Bill for private health care

You would like to refer Bill to a podiatric surgeon regarding surgical options for the treatment of his bunions which are now extremely painful. This type of consultation is not available locally on the NHS. It would therefore be necessary to be seen by a private practice. Bill is unable to afford the consultation fee, or the costs of any subsequent surgery. He does not have any private medical insurance to cover the cost. How would you approach this situation, particularly given that Bill has strongly held beliefs about private medicine?

This scenario presents the podiatrist with a professional dilemma. It is a common reaction for professionals to be judgemental about how patients should prioritise their financial expenditure. It is clear that by curtailing his smoking and alcohol intake, Bill may be able to afford the necessary orthosis in a relatively short space of time. However, he is most reluctant to spend his money on private health care, believing that the NHS should provide him with any necessary treatment. In addition, he maintains that being a regular in his local pub represents 'his only pleasure'.

This problem reflects an important principle in understanding health-related behaviour. Risk to health is not always perceived as a deterrent to potentially damaging behaviours. It is highly improbable that Bill is unaware of the risks that smoking and excessive drinking carry to his health. Many studies have demonstrated high levels of awareness of the risk of tobacco use amongst smokers (Altman *et al.*, 1996; Sasco and Kleihues, 1999; Vora *et al.*, 2000). In fact, some research has shown that smokers may even overestimate the risks they run of developing certain diseases, such as lung cancer (Sutton, 1998).

However, Bill considers that these risks are worth taking, because of the pleasure that he derives from his social life. Moreover, for many people immediate fulfilment is seen as preferable to benefits which are only accrued after a prolonged period.

The podiatrist has to make a decision as to whether to attempt to persuade Bill to change his behaviour in order that he can afford the surgery. Alternatively, it may be more appropriate simply to recognise Bill's needs while accepting that many patients may have values that are different from those of health professionals.

This is a matter for professional judgement and discretion, which can only be addressed adequately by understanding the patient as a whole and respecting and acknowledging his social identity, values and choices.

Challenge 2: How does the manner in which Bill is treated by his work colleagues influence his health and choices?

It is clearly established that inequalities in social status impact on physical health. However, it is equally important to appreciate that the British class system can be particularly destructive in terms of people's emotional health and sense of well-being.

People in lower socio-economic groups are systematically made to feel disempowered and less valuable than those in higher socio-economic groups (Hunter and Killoran, 2004). Conversely, people in higher socio-economic groups have their own sets of social constraints within which they are expected to conform. In Bill's case, the offhand treatment he receives from his employers and the parents serves to foster his resentment against professionals in general. It is therefore possible that he will be less receptive to the podiatrist's well-meaning attempts to alter his smoking and drinking habits. In order to change his behaviour, it is essential that Bill perceives any such change as being his choice rather than something that is imposed on him. The podiatrist needs to understand this and must develop a relationship of mutual trust and respect. The podiatrist's task is complete when he/she is assured that Bill is in receipt of all appropriate information in order to make an informed choice. However, Bill's choice may be at variance with that of the podiatrist, and this must ultimately be accepted. Any attempt to change Bill's behaviour will rely heavily on the podiatrist possessing good communication skills, which will underpin all podiatric practice.

Summary of important health psychology

It is well established that substantial inequalities in health status are independently related to social status. People in lower socio-economic groups suffer from poorer health and have higher rates of mortality than do people in higher socio-economic groups. This effect is dependent upon *differences* in affluence rather than absolute measures of wealth. Western class systems equate social and financial position with intrinsic personal worth. Relative poverty thus results in the exclusion of less privileged people from complete participation in society.

Implications for podiatric management

On the face of it, Bill's podiatric problems will require assessment and probably a diagnosis of plantar fasciitis arising from the cavoid foot shape and his increased weight. However, the holistic approach to Bill's foot problems must also be considered and, as previously mentioned, perhaps the greatest challenge to the podiatrist in his management is the behavioural change required to enable Bill to be pain-free. It may be perfectly possible to relieve Bill's symptoms with the use of orthoses; however, considering all the contributory factors, simply using mechanical devices may be insufficient. In addition, Bill's footwear must be able to accommodate any device provided and consideration for shoe style will be important. Bill may require non-steroidal anti-inflammatory drugs (NSAIDs) or even steroid injections.

The podiatrist must negotiate with Bill a commitment to smoking cessation and to improvements in his diet. It may be that Bill finds it odd that someone advising on his feet should start to talk about more general health-related issues, and the podiatrist should have available the contacts for smoking cessation classes and referral pathways to dietetic services. Further assessment of Bill's general health may also be necessary, especially as he is at greater risk of type 2 diabetes and cardiovascular disease. Perhaps a clue to his potential development of diabetes is that he reports that his feet have not always been quite so highly arched and that the associated claw toes appear to be becoming more pronounced.

Chapter 12

Working with patients who have a dual diagnosis

Remember when you were young, you shone like the sun . . .
Now there's a look in your eyes, like black holes in the sky.
Roger Waters

Matthew Johnson is a 32-year-old man. Following the death of his father when Matthew was in his early teens, he was brought up by his mother. An only child, Matthew did not make friends easily at school, and was somewhat introspective, particularly as an adolescent. He has always described himself as 'a bit of a loner', preferring his own company to that of others. This tendency served to reinforce his insular reputation and some of his schoolmates considered him 'a little odd'. When he was 19 years of age, Matthew joined the British Army. Opportunities to travel, combined with the offer of learning a practical trade provided an attractive future. Moreover, the comradeship and sense of belonging that the armed forces offers its members represented an extended family in which Matthew felt secure; the routine and highly structured environment of the army gave him a sense of order and permanence that he had felt lacking for many years.

Matthew flourished in military life until around four years ago, when he was sent to serve a tour of duty in Iraq. Matthew was horrified by the scenes he witnessed and had severe doubts about the rightness of his actions. At first, he became increasingly withdrawn and asocial. Later, he expressed the belief that he was being watched constantly, and finally admitted to the medical officer that he heard voices telling him to harm himself. Matthew's condition worsened and when he was eventually discharged from the Army on medical grounds, he found the return to civilian life especially difficult.

With no extended family and little appropriate resettlement advice, his occasional use of marijuana became more regular. As so frequently happens, this aggravated his pre-existing mental health problems and his hallucinatory symptoms increased.

From time to time, Matthew disappeared from home and lived rough on the streets. He would be subsequently returned by the police in a disturbed state, having succumbed to heroin and crack cocaine. By now, Matthew's life was a series of chaotic experiences with many statutory and voluntary agencies involved in his care.

Podiatric presentation

Matthew has been referred to the podiatry clinic by his general practitioner. Matthew appears dishevelled and unkempt. His clothing is dirty and his hair appears not to have been washed for several weeks. On examination, Matthew's feet are dirty, and there is evidence of a long-standing fungal infection. It is evident that his nails have not been cut for a long period. Some have overgrown and penetrated the soft tissues of the lesser digits; others have broken off, leaving open wounds which exhibit signs of infection. On his left big toe, he has an Ostlers' nail (onychogryphosis with accompanying sepsis).

Relevant psychological theory

Schizophrenia is a psychotic illness that affects just over 1% of the UK population. Onset is usually in late adolescence or early adulthood. The condition affects men and women equally. There is a genetic link to the illness, by which an individual with one parent with schizophrenia carries a risk of 14% of developing symptoms. If both parents have schizophrenia, the likelihood of their child developing the condition is 46%. The precise causation of the illness is not certain, but a number of hypotheses have been suggested. The most influential of these is the so-called Dopamine Hypothesis (Seeman et al., 1976). It has long been known that most antipsychotic drugs block dopamine receptors, and that neuroleptic potency is directly proportional to receptor blocking potency. Schizophrenic symptoms can be precipitated by drugs such as amphetamines, which are known to increase dopaminergic activity. Moreover, post-mortem studies have shown excessive dopamine concentrations in the brains of people who have suffered from schizophrenia. In addition, patients with schizophrenia often show electroencephalographic and brain scan abnormalities. Schizophrenia is often associated with temporal lobe epilepsy, birth complications, winter births and maternal viral infections in pregnancy (Kohler et al., 2001).

Treatment for schizophrenia primarily involves drug therapy, and the complexity of the illness often results in patients presenting with complex drug regimes. The major group of medicines employed are known as *neuroleptics*, or antipsychotic agents. These include drugs that have been used for many years, such as chlorpromazine and haloperidol, together with relatively newer preparations such as clozapine and rispiridol. All these drugs can be effective in reducing the occurrence of severe symptoms, such as hallucinations and delusions, but have unpleasant side effects, such as weight gain, dry mouth and pseudo-parkinsonian symptoms (muscle rigidity, altered gait and tremors). Anti-parkinsonian medications are often prescribed in an attempt to counteract these symptoms, but are often only partially successful in doing so. In addition, many people with schizophrenia experience depressive symptoms which may be concurrently treated with antidepressants such as citalopram, fluoxetine and amitriptyline. *Talking therapies*, such as cognitive behavioural therapy, have become increasingly important in the treatment of schizophrenia. While the body of evidence for their effectiveness is increasing, the number of trained therapists in the NHS remains limited at the time of writing.

Schizophrenia is *episodic* in nature: some patients experience only one episode and then make a complete recovery, whilst others experience multiple psychotic episodes throughout their lives. The illness often runs a chronic course and can leave residual psychiatric symptoms and impaired social functioning. In its active phase, the illness often begins with the affected person experiencing delusions. Delusions are fixed, false beliefs which cannot be influenced by rational argument. Such beliefs may involve grandiose ideas, but more typically are characterised by feelings of unworthiness and guilt. Many people who suffer from schizophrenia believe that they are persecuted, watched or under surveillance by individuals, organisations or agencies. Later, many sufferers experience hallucinations and multiple disturbances of mental processes.

Hallucinations are sensory experiences for which there is no obvious cause. Most commonly, sufferers experience auditory hallucinations, during which sounds, usually voices, are heard. These voices are occasionally pleasant or amusing, and may result in the patient smiling or laughing for no apparent reason. Far more commonly, however, the voices may be critical, threatening or abusive (Andreasen *et al.*, 1995). Sometimes the voices may instruct the person to harm or kill themselves. Other forms of hallucination include seeing objects, people or scenes that do not exist, while still other sufferers describe tactile experiences, in which they experience the sensation of objects, often insects, crawling over or beneath their skin. Less commonly, some people with schizophrenia experience strange tastes or can smell odours which others do not.

It must be emphasised that although there is no obvious cause for the sensations that people with schizophrenia report, the experiences themselves are utterly realistic to the sufferer. Voices, for example, are heard as clearly and realistically as actual voices; beliefs of persecution are as firmly held and considered as justified as any other. The effect that these experiences have on most people is extremely frightening. During hallucinatory phases, sufferers may display agitation, excitability or aggression in response to the things that they see, hear or feel. Speech may become unintelligible.

Initially, relatives and friends notice that the individual has become socially withdrawn, and a loss of motivation is seen. A 'blunting' of emotions is common, and the sufferer may show little interest in activities of any kind, appearing indifferent to events, whether good or bad. Loss of concentration and impairment of memory is often reported, and for this reason the condition may first manifest itself as a deterioration of school work, when occurring in young people.

Importantly for Matthew, around 50% of patients display pre-morbid personality symptoms (Peralta *et al.*, 1991) known as *schizoid* features; the social isolation and eccentricity shown by Matthew as a teenager are very common in young adults who go on to experience schizophrenic symptoms. Family dynamics are less widely held to be an aetiological factor, but some authors suggest that critical, overly involved parents with high levels of *expressed emotion* may influence the onset of symptoms in vulnerable individuals. Perhaps most pertinent for Matthew, traumatic life events may trigger acute episodes.

Depression is extremely common among people with schizophrenia. This is particularly the case during the phase of the illness in which recovery is beginning to occur. As the sufferer becomes more aware of their condition and cognitive functioning returns, many people with schizophrenia become acutely aware of the prognosis of their illness, and suicide attempts are common. In order to cope with the psychological pain involved, many people with schizophrenia misuse alcohol or drugs. Such patients are often said to have a *dual diagnosis*, which is estimated to affect around 30% to 50% of people with schizophrenia (Dixon, 1999).

Factors influencing Matthew's behaviour

Perhaps the overriding difficulty facing people with any severe mental health problem is the attitudes and reactions of other people towards them. There is widespread prejudice against mental illness, which is exacerbated by the popular press. Schizophrenia is frequently associated (wrongly) with violence and unpredictable behaviour, and people suffering from schizophrenia are commonly viewed with suspicion and distrust. In fact, such attitudes are groundless. The vast majority of violent crime is committed by people with no history of mental illness whatsoever. By contrast, people with schizophrenia are much more likely to be a danger to themselves, either through neglect or in response to accusatory hallucinations or depression. Rates of suicide and attempted suicide are very high among individuals suffering from schizophrenia (Siris, 2001).

Two important studies have investigated the relationship between homelessness and previous service in the armed forces (Randall and Brown, 1994; Gunner and Knott, 1997). It was found that people who had previously served in the armed forces represent 30% of homeless people living in hostels, day centres and using soup runs, and made up 22% of homeless people surveyed in London on a single night. Only 8% of these people had served as part of National Service; 86% having joined voluntarily. There is a relationship between length of service in the military and the likelihood of becoming homeless. In 1994, ex-service personnel who had up to three years' service made up 19% of homeless people. Thirty per cent had served for three to six years and 51% had served over six years. Seventy-eight per cent of service personnel leaving the service do so because they have reached the end of their contract, rather than for reasons of health, disciplinary procedures or other factors. The detrimental effects of military service appear to be most pronounced among soldiers, rather than individuals from the air force or the navy.

In our view, this clearly demonstrates that the longer the period of service, the greater the risk of being unable to move back into civilian life. It is also likely that these startling figures may be related to the nature of military life. The military regime is highly regulated, highly hierarchical and offers little by way of individual choice. Immediate, unquestioning obedience to orders, even in relation to acts which may run contrary to an individual's nature, is both demanded and considered normal. These features may well be responsible for the common difficulties experienced by ex-service personnel attempting to integrate back into civilian society.

Challenge 1: What sort of approach should the podiatrist adopt when working with Matthew?

Acceptance, empathy and a non-judgemental approach are essential in Matthew's care. Whilst such a statement is easy to make, it requires the podiatrist to reconsider what he or she may view as being normal. Alcohol or drugs (or both) are commonly used by people with schizophrenia in order to blunt the pain and distress that both their immediate symptoms and their prognosis create, and their use must not be seen as deviant or irresponsible. Drug and alcohol use is an unfortunate, but arguably inevitable, consequence of the psychological suffering experienced by people with severe mental health problems.

Simple acts of care can be enormously helpful for people with schizophrenia. Personal hygiene, nail care and grooming are often neglected because of the overriding effects of hallucinations or the sense of worthlessness brought about by delusions and depression.

Challenge 2: How will Matthew's behaviour change when he is experiencing an active episode of schizophrenia?

During an acute episode of schizophrenia, sufferers may feel that their minds are being bombarded from all directions by ideas, questions and commands. They may feel too overwhelmed to consider even minor problems. People with schizophrenia may use words that sound like nonsense to others. If you cannot be understood, you should try to express your interest and concern in other ways; good non-verbal communication skills are extremely important. The podiatrist should try to be as supportive and understanding as possible, and to speak in a calm, clear and straightforward manner. People with schizophrenia are usually aware of what is going on around them, even if they appear not to be listening.

Who will be involved in supporting Matthew?

For most people who have schizophrenia, taking a prescribed medication regularly is crucial to their ongoing health. The lack of ambition and reduced capacity for self-care that are characteristic of schizophrenia, often combined with delusory beliefs, frequently result in poor concordance with medication regimes as will as with prescribed exercises or other treatment. Unless supported by others, all forms of treatment are likely to be haphazard, and effective communication with other professionals involved with Matthew's care is essential. Generally, a key worker (often a community mental health nurse) will have been assigned to an individual, but this is not always the case. Homelessness is very common among people with severe mental health problems (see Chapter 17), and the podiatrist may be one of the few professionals in contact.

Support and encouragement to take medication regularly can make a vital difference. To do this, the podiatrist needs to gain Matthew's trust and confidence as an individual, rather than simply as a health professional. Expressions of a suicidal nature *must* be treated seriously, even if they are couched in terms or ideas that seem bizarre.

Helping people with schizophrenia to stay as healthy as possible takes a team – family, friends, health care professionals, support groups – working together, over the long term. Caring for a person with a schizophrenic illness is exhausting, stressful and emotionally draining. As a result, family members and carers commonly neglect to take proper care of themselves. They may give up their own activities and become isolated from their friends and colleagues. Their stress can lead to sleeping problems, exhaustion and constant irritability. Carers may often accompany patients such a Matthew, and empathy, care and understanding are essential in meeting their needs as well as those of the patient. A positive outcome, in which a person with schizophrenia is enabled to remain stable while living and functioning in the community, makes the effort very worthwhile.

Implications for podiatric management

Matthew's initial podiatric treatment is relatively straightforward and likely to consist of the reduction of the long, thickened toenails and wound care. However, his situation militates against maintaining his foot health. He will almost certainly be ineligible for routine podiatric state-funded provision because of his relatively young age and the lack of a complicating, systemic disease. However, some services may have acute or severe mental health conditions as part of their access criteria for funded services. Additionally, his straitened financial position is such that he is highly unlikely to seek treatment in the private sector; yet the likelihood of his acquiring further multiple infections is high as a result of his living and social circumstances. It may be possible, however, that suitable routine care may be available through the voluntary sector, and it is therefore imperative that the podiatrist is familiar with such provision in the area in which he/she practises. Moreover, it is of great value in clinical practice to establish a working relationship with a wide range of agencies within both statutory independent and voluntary sectors.

Matthew is typical of patients who have complex needs, and the podiatrist should be able to use his contact with podiatric services opportunistically in order to facilitate access to appropriate care agencies.

Postscript

The real 'Matthew Johnson' suffered from schizophrenia and was dependent on heroin and crack cocaine for several years. Matthew was severely depressed by his symptoms and was acutely aware of his poor prognosis. He disappeared one evening and was discovered several days later, having committed suicide. He was constantly and bravely supported by his mother throughout his illness and complex difficulties. We are very grateful to his mother for her assistance in the writing of this chapter.

Chapter 13

Complex interactions illustrating the need for good interpersonal and communication skills

How inimitably graceful children are in general before they learn to dance!

Samuel Taylor Coleridge

Olivia Saunders presents the podiatrist with a complex interaction which involves: a professional, a child and the child's parents. This situation is explored and the importance of good interpersonal and communication skills highlighted. The need for appropriate health promotion approaches is also discussed.

Olivia is an eight-year-old ballet dancer who has been having ballet lessons since she was three years of age. She has always loved dancing and already aspires to be a professional dancer. Her immediate ambition is to audition, as soon as possible, for a scholarship to the Royal Ballet School. She has worked hard at her ballet exams and has always passed with high marks and honours.

Olivia is a pretty, young girl with a typical slim ballerina's physique. She is elegant and has poise with an air of determination and commitment when talking about her chosen career as a professional dancer. She is the only daughter of Mr and Mrs Saunders, who support their daughter, and are very keen to help her to fulfil her ambition.

Olivia is pressuring her parents to allow her to start to wear pointe shoes (ballet shoes with wooden blocks in the toes), even though she knows she is too young. She knows that she should really wait until she reaches menarche but feels that wearing pointe will give her the edge over her peers. Olivia thinks that starting to wear pointe shoes will help her to achieve her goal of studying at the Royal Ballet School. Her ballet teacher, Miss Turner, would be very proud of Olivia if she were successful in achieving a scholarship, and would see it as a direct reflection of her teaching ability. Miss Turner turned to teaching ballet after a disappointing career in the *corps de ballet* but always felt that her talents should have been recognised, and that she was worthy of being a principal ballerina. She hopes to see Olivia have the acclaim that she never received. Mr and Mrs Saunders are influenced by the opinions of people they consider to be more expert than themselves. They have read that dancers should not be wearing pointe shoes as early as eight years old, and need to be reassured that this is safe and appropriate before agreeing to Olivia's wishes. On the one hand, they would like to accede to Olivia's demands but, on the other, they are concerned for her current and future health and welfare. Consequently, they have decided to seek impartial professional advice.

Factors influencing Olivia's behaviour

Children do not think issues through in the same way as adults. Their thinking is simpler than adults, and it is difficult for them to predict how an event or behaviour today may impact on tomorrow.

It is important to recognise that Olivia is very competitive and extremely motivated. Motivation is highly relevant to the achievement of the goals being pursued, to the intensity of the behaviour and to the persistence in the behaviour. There are various early theories which consider factors such as instinct, needs and drives, which are now considered somewhat limited, for example Maslow (1954, 1970) posited the existence of a 'hierarchy of needs' which must be met for an individual to survive and to develop, that is shelter, food etc. These 'needs' provide motivational sources for behaviour. One aspect of motivation is the goal, and the need of the individual to achieve that goal (Locke, 1968). Locke suggests that there is a linear relationship between goal difficulty and level of performance. In Olivia's case, her goal is very difficult to achieve and will require high levels of performance, which may result in damage to her health.

Reinforcement is a technique that the podiatrist may employ with Olivia. Health professionals should provide positive reinforcement for behaviours that are most likely to help the patient achieve their goals. Patients seek both verbal and non-verbal positive feedback. Feedback expresses either approval of the desired behaviour or disapproval of maladaptive behaviour.

Another approach to consider is the use of *positive role models*. Identification with a positive role model can demonstrate positive health values and outcomes. Children who have positive role models around them, or who identify with positive role models, are more likely to choose the same healthy behaviours. This may in turn provide a positive self-image which remains with the child throughout life (Ikeda and Naworski, 1992).

Olivia needs to be aware that she may become subject to ankle and foot injury as a result of excessive training. Acute traumatic injuries are common in ballet dancers (MacIntyre and Joy, 2000). Where there is incomplete rehabilitation, these may often develop into repeated injuries.

The performance demands of ballet are very high and can be compared to those made of athletes. It is the athletic demands of dance choreography that can place the dancer at risk for injuries of which foot injuries are common. In fact, 15–20% of dance injuries involve the foot. Moreover, the presence of chronic injuries predominates owing to the repetitive impact loading of the dancer's foot on a relatively hard dance floor.

The ballet shoe is only a thin slipper made from satin and ribbon. The shock-absorbing mechanism provided is through the presence of a stiff cardboard midsole, cotton insole and stiff cardboard outsole. The tip of the shoe is glued canvas to allow dancers to achieve the full *pointe*. These mechanisms do not reduce the impact of the forces incurred, which are ultimately absorbed by the lower extremities. The failure to effectively and efficiently absorb these forces can lead to injury to structures about the foot. Factors that can contribute to this ineffective absorption of energy include anatomic variation, improper technique and, in some cases, fatigue.

Turnout of the hip, or maximum external rotation, is the single most important anatomic factor in classical ballet. There are five basic positions in ballet, each of which involves maximum external rotation of the hip, and all ballet movements begin or end with one of these positions. Dancers who are able to adopt maximum external rotation may be demonstrating ligamentous laxity in order to achieve this position. Those dancers who have a less marked 'natural' turnout at the hip may compensate by forcing external rotation at the knee or the foot and ankle joints, thereby incurring the potential for injury.

Some dancers have inadequate external rotation at the hip and so employ a technique called *rolling in*, which is the equivalent of excessive pronation. This movement involves eversion of the hindfoot with forced pronation of the midfoot and forefoot. Such positioning can result in excessive strain on the medial structures of the foot and ankle, and can lead to chronic injuries. Other injuries can occur from foot shapes such as a cavus foot, with its inherent rigid midtarsal joint. The cavus foot is not designed to absorb energy and is especially vulnerable to ligamentous strain, fasciitis and stress fractures.

Injuries may also occur when the ballet shoes have worn out; this is when the shoe becomes too soft to be able to supports them *en pointe*. At this point the shoe can collapse, resulting in the dancer's foot rolling over when *en pointe*.

The dance surface is another potential source of injury. Dance surfaces must provide adequate shock absorption yet be firm enough to provide sufficient energy return to the dancer to enhance performance and reduce fatigue. Surfaces that are too firm with little or no give may lead to early muscular fatigue because the musculoskeletal system of the lower extremities must act to absorb most of the shock. Where there is inadequate shock absorption, stress fractures may occur. Conversely, if a dance surface is too soft, there will be adequate absorption but inadequate energy return to the dancer, thus requiring considerably more effort to perform the desired movements. This can result in fatigue and thence injury.

A common complaint in adolescent ballet dances is *epiphysitis*. Epiphysitis occurs due to the first metatarsalphalangeal joint being subjected to extensive dorsiflexion. The joint is not normally exposed to such demands and responds by moulding the growing epiphysis. Epiphysitis is characterised by tenderness, inflammation and pain with activity and is relieved by rest. The condition tends to recur, but disappears when the epiphysis fuses at maturity.

Cuboid subluxations in females differ from those occurring in males (Marshall and Hamilton, 1992; MacIntyre and Joy, 2000). In men, cuboid dislocations are usually acute and occur as a result of a series of jumps (in ballet terms, a *bravura* variation) when the foot is repeatedly pronated under force. A sequence of movements, such as the *releves* (a repetitive movement from foot flat to balancing on the tips of their toes, and back again) can result in overuse syndrome. Dancers moving from foot flat to *full pointe* (on tips of their toes) may find remaining in the full pointe position difficult and consequently balance on the dorsal surface of the metatarsal heads. In addition, the resultant alterations of direction and force applied to the foot during repetitive movements such as 'releves' will contribute to reduced joint stability. The repetitive nature of ballet movements can result in *hypermobility*, which in turn predisposes dancers to cuboid dislocations (Marshall and Hamilton, 1992; MacIntyre and Joy, 2000). Whilst it is possible for females to dislocate the cuboid, subluxation of the cuboid is more common, and a result of overuse, and may become part of an overuse syndrome.

Ligamentous laxity is considered to be a further factor in the cause of dance injury (Newell and Woodie, 1981; Blakeslee and Morris, 1987; Marshall and Hamilton, 1992; MacIntyre and Joy, 2000). Most ballet dancers subject their joints to extreme ranges of motion in order to perform certain movements, thereby increasing the likelihood of injury (Newell and Woodie, 1981; Blakeslee and Morris, 1987; Marshall and Hamilton, 1992; MacIntyre and Joy, 2000).

Comprehensive assessment, diagnosis and management of acute injuries are required to prevent injuries such as ligament tears and tendon pathologies from becoming chronic. As part of management, attention should be paid to nutrition in order to both facilitate the healing of existing injuries and to prevent the possible development of conditions such as osteoporosis. Osteoporosis is considered in more detail in Chapter 5. Without consideration of the psychological factors associated with injury, pain perception and concordance with treatment, successful rehabilitation may be limited.

Great care should be exercised when designing a training regime suitable for prepubescent children. Growth periods are difficult to identify, and are of uncertain duration. Therefore, any undue pressure should not be placed on the long bones when epiphyseal closure may not have taken place. Moreover, sub-maximal muscle strength training is more appropriate to the growing child. This involves the use of training which focuses on the trunk, and is considered to provide flexibility, balance and coordination, which are fundamental to remaining injury free (Phillips, 1999). Such a training regime is preferable to the early use of pointe shoes, and the podiatrist should suggest this approach to Olivia and her parents.

The presence of painful skin lesions, for example corns, and in particular interdigital lesions, often results in dancers suspending their training regime. Golomer and Chatellier (1990) found that the number of skin lesions is correlated to the degree of tightness of the pointe shoe: the tighter the shoe, the more skin lesions. Palliative podiatric treatment, that is the reduction of the painful corns, will allow dancers to return to their training schedule; however, it is almost inevitable that the lesions will recur and disrupt training once again.

In addition to skin, other soft-tissue structures, such as tendons, bursae and fascia, may be injured as a consequence of excessive and repeated stress. Finally, joint injury may result in longer periods of rehabilitation, with recurring episodes of injury responsible for chronic joint disease leading, in the long term, to arthritis.

It is a truism, but important, to consider that the tips of the toes were never intended to support the entire body's weight, and that such an abnormal posture will inevitably result in pain and injury.

Challenge 1: What are the possible motivations for Olivia's wish to wear pointe shoes?

Such motivations may include:

■ competitiveness
■ a desire to be 'grown-up'

- a desire and/need to be the first in her group to achieve desired goals
- the expected inability of Olivia, a child, to assess the long-term effects of her current behaviour
- Olivia's desire to please her dance teacher.

You should consider this challenge and reflect on how you would feel if asked to offer an opinion regarding the wisdom of Mr and Mrs Saunders allowing Olivia to wear pointe shoes. It is likely that what you have to say will not be what Olivia wishes to hear, and she may resent your involvement. You will have to consider how you will deliver this information in a way that will be acceptable to Olivia.

Challenge 2: How can you enable Olivia and her parents to acknowledge the benefits of *not* using pointe ballet shoes?

The information which Olivia requires includes the importance from both a developmental and a foot health perspective, that she does not wear pointe ballet shoes until at least her menarche. Structurally, her feet are not yet strong enough to be able to deal with the stresses of using pointe shoes and so she will have a greater chance of developing toe deformities.

A useful approach to health promotion may involve the following:

- Exploring Olivia's beliefs about early pointe work.
- Reinforcing any positive attitudes she may have.
- Discussing myths about and attitudes towards dance.
- Exploring with Olivia and her parents the perceived costs and benefits of wearing pointe shoes.
- Providing reliable information to assist the family to make informed choices.
- Devising a negotiated plan of action.
- Monitoring Olivia's progress.

The health education and promotion approach could include the use of strengthening exercises that would prepare Olivia for the time when she reaches a suitable age to wear pointe shoes. If possible, alternatives to wearing pointe shoes should be suggested. This approach may provide different positive reinforcements for Olivia. It will also provide Mr and Mrs Saunders with an explanation of the short- and long-term costs and benefits if Olivia chooses to dances in pointe shoes early.

Summary of important health psychology

It is important that the podiatrist understands the complex interactions which can occur between a professional, a child and the child's parent(s). Well-developed interpersonal and communication skills are essential to ensuring a successful outcome in a situation such as this. An understanding of effective health promotion is important in order to design strategies that will enable Olivia to prevent the development of injuries.

Implications for podiatric management

The absence of symptoms makes the podiatric management of this case different from most podiatric consultations. It is the convention in podiatric practice that foot complaints are analysed, health assessed and some form of treatment plan implemented. In this case, there are no symptoms, and the podiatrist's familiar working practices must be put to one side. Successful management for Olivia centres on arriving at an understanding with both Olivia and her parents about the implications of her ambition to move into pointe shoes too soon. Perhaps consideration of developmental timelines may help this understanding, and a commitment to monitor Olivia's progress through her growth and development in association with her dancing teachers would be useful. Exercise, for example swimming, that do not require as much impact as dancing may also be appropriate to strengthen muscles around joints.

Chapter 14

The importance of confidentiality and negotiating informed consent

It is tact that is golden, not silence.
Samuel Butler

Peter Brennan is a patient with complex needs. Peter's treatment and management require the podiatrist to recognise the importance of confidentiality between professional disciplines and the need to negotiate informed consent. The complex nature of this case will require the podiatrist to consider how best to deal with sensitive and confidential material.

Peter is 35 years old. He is a small man, approximately 1 m 7 cm tall and weighs about 60 kg. Peter has a serious face, dark-coloured eyes, dark-brown hair and looks slightly older than his actual age. He is employed as a social worker by the local authority, in a senior position. Apart from his podiatric condition, he seems fit and well, with a cheerful, open manner. As part of taking his history, you ask him whether he is taking any form of medication. Peter replies that he has been on continuous combined therapy since being diagnosed as HIV positive three years ago.

He has remained well throughout this period and is in regular contact with local HIV services. While he is direct about his condition in the context of his treatment, Peter does not make his HIV status known generally. Peter is single and lives alone in a flat in a pleasant part of the town. He has a sister, who lives at the other end of the country. Peter's parents are both alive and well but are both elderly; his relationship with them is good.

Podiatric presentation

Peter presents with multiple warts on the plantar surface of his feet. You want to use an antiviral, which is a prescription-only medicine, and it will therefore be necessary for you to contact Peter's GP. It is extremely important that Peter's lesions are kept free from possible infection following treatment. Patients who are immunosuppressed will be more susceptible to secondary infections, which they will be less able to overcome.

Clearly, Peter's HIV status presents a number of problems in relation to infection control. These may be usefully considered, first, in relation to himself and, second, in relation to those professionals providing his treatment. Patients whose immune systems are compromised for any reason, including HIV infection, are much more susceptible to secondary infections and this must be taken into consideration when considering Peter's treatment regime.

Human immune deficiency virus

This is a viral infection which is caused by the human immunodeficiency virus (HIV) that gradually destroys the immune system.

Causes and risks

Acute HIV infection may be associated with symptoms resembling mononucleosis or the flu within two to four weeks of exposure. HIV sero-conversion (converting from HIV negative to HIV positive) occurs within three months of exposure.

People who become infected with HIV may have no symptoms for up to 10 years, but they can still transmit the infection to others. Meanwhile, their immune system gradually weakens until they are diagnosed with AIDS. Acute HIV infection progresses over time to asymptomatic HIV infection and then to early symptomatic HIV infection and, later, to AIDS.

HIV infection may be passed through the maternal bloodstream to the foetus, resulting in the baby being HIV positive when born. HIV may also be transmitted by contact with infected blood, and frequently occurs when intravenous drug users share injecting equipment. More commonly, HIV is transmitted sexually. Although the infection was first noticed in the 1980s among gay men, heterosexually transmitted HIV infection is now much more common and is increasing rapidly.

Most individuals infected with HIV will progress to AIDS if not treated. However, there is a very small subset of patients who develop AIDS very slowly, or never at all. These patients are called *non-progressors*.

Acquired immune deficiency syndrome

AIDS stands for acquired immune deficiency syndrome. AIDS is caused by the human immunodeficiency virus (HIV). AIDS is characterised by the progressively immunocompromised state of the infected individual (Soltani *et al.*, 1996). Disease progression is monitored by a continuous decrease in peripheral blood CD4+ T lymphocytes, which are targeted by HIV infection. These cells play an important role in the immune system, hence the gradual loss of the patient's immune system. AIDS is the final and most serious stage of HIV disease, in which the signs and symptoms of severe immunodeficiency have developed.

Cutaneous podiatric implications

The course of HIV can have a devastating effect on lower-limb mobility and function, and the role of the podiatrist may be fundamental to the care team (McReynolds, 1995). Podiatrists will be particularly aware of the opportunistic infections occurring as a result of cell-mediated and humoral immunodeficiency. The most common infections are caused by staphylococcus aureus, streptococcus A, C and G and ulcers infected with Pseudomonas auruginosa (Memar *et al.*, 1995). Furthermore, in the early stages of the disease tinea pedis (fungal infections) and verrucae are more common. Smith *et al.* (1994) report that verrucae appeared to become more diffuse and resilient to treatment as the disease progressed. Other complications include increased risk of cutaneous epidermal and melanotic malignancies, including Kaposi's sarcoma. Non-infectious disorders include inflammatory disorders, pruritus, hypersensitivities, dryness and dermatoses.

Challenge 1: What are the important issues concerning Peter's psychological care?

Psychological care

It is very important to appreciate that adequate protection against accidental infection with HIV is afforded by routine procedures, often described as *universal precautions*. Such procedures are those which should be taken with all patients: the podiatrist does not need to take any other specific precautions when treating a patient who is known to be HIV positive. In Peter's case, any of the available treatments may involve the use of debridement, which could result in loss of some blood or serous fluid. However, such clinical waste should always be treated with appropriate care because many patients may be carrying blood-borne diseases of which they are unaware, and some of which (for example hepatitis) are far more contagious than the HIV virus. Much unnecessary fear and misunderstanding continues to exist with regard to HIV transmission, even amongst health professionals. Such misunderstanding may easily manifest in levels of caution which are inappropriate and which can serve to distance still further patients who already experience prejudice and alienation as a result of earlier reactions to their condition.

Nevertheless, there are important issues for the podiatrist concerning Peter's treatment. It must be recognised that the consideration of the route by which Peter acquired the virus is outside the professional boundaries of podiatric practice and is irrelevant to his podiatric treatment. All podiatrists, like other health professionals, have a *duty of care*, which requires them to provide treatment to the best of their ability. In order to achieve this with all patients, it is insufficient for the podiatrist to assume that their duty of care negates any discriminatory feelings they may hold. There will be times when patients present information that is contrary to the podiatrist's beliefs or culture. It is necessary for the podiatrist to recognise that such differences will occur and to recognise that all people are free to behave and express themselves in ways that are appropriate for them. It is also very important for practitioners to recognise their own professional boundaries and not to attempt to address issues that are outside their scope of practice and competence. It is therefore necessary for all health professionals to examine their own attitudes towards complex issues such as drug use and sexuality in relation to their own professional practice.

The need for confidentiality is particularly important in Peter's treatment. While confidentiality is an essential characteristic of all patient–therapist interactions, the emotive response sometimes generated by HIV-related issues has specific implications for his welfare. Peter works in the public sector in a sensitive position, which is often the subject of criticism and stereotyping (Pietroni, 1991). Confidentiality is a fundamental right of all patients and, in Peter's case, any unauthorised disclosure of his status could be extremely damaging.

However, you will need to contact Peter's GP for prescription of the antiviral medication and possible onward referral to dermatology. This may raise issues of confidentiality because the GP may not necessarily be aware of Peter's HIV status. It will be necessary to negotiate permission for this dialogue.

Challenge 2: What are Peter's particular needs in relation to his podiatric condition?

James *et al.* (2001) show that patients taking combination therapy are more prone to onychocryptosis, or in-growing toenails. They found that, out of a group of 74 patients taking indinavir and retinovir, five patients (6.8%) were suffering from onychocryptosis involving the big toe. Onychocryptosis is often associated with paronychia (inflammation of the skin surrounding the nails), which may lead to infection. Whilst such infections are easily treated in most patients, people with HIV have suppressed immune systems and so minor infections can become much more serious in a short space of time. It is therefore very important that any signs of infection are dealt with without delay.

James *et al.* (2001) stress that as combination therapy becomes more widely used, complications such as in-growing toenails are more likely to become more common. The authors further recommend that all patients taking combination therapy should have their hands and feet examined regularly.

Summary of important health psychology

The podiatrist should be aware of the possibility of Peter being anxious or depressed as a result of his general condition. It is likely that Peter will respond best to an empathetic, non-judgemental communication style. Of great importance is the development of trust within the relationship in order that Peter is assured that the podiatrist will abide by agreed principles and will practise ethically, maintaining confidentiality.

Implications for podiatric management

There are four key issues in relation to Peter's podiatric treatment and management. First, that the spread of HIV infection is adequately controlled by the use of universal precautions and no special procedures are required over and above those of normal hygiene and cross-infection control protocols. It maybe wise, however, to see Peter at the end of a clinical session, when decontamination of the environment can take place. It is the duty of the podiatrist to abide by the latest decontamination and sterilisation regulations and procedures. Details of these are available from the local infection control department and on health and safety websites. Compliance with national legislation is vital.

Second, it is important for the podiatrist to recognise his/her professional competence in relation to Peter's infection. Third, confidentiality is an essential part of the care of any patient but the nature of Peter's condition brings the need for confidentiality into sharper focus.

Finally, it is very important when treating patients who are immuno-suppressed in any way to examine thoroughly for signs of infections or reported symptoms of general malaise so that appropriate treatment can be instigated at the earliest opportunity.

Chapter 15

Safety and independence: considerations when dealing with early-stage dementia

Before you contradict an old man, my fair friend, you should endeavour to understand him.

George Santayana

Rose Stuart is a slightly built widowed lady aged 78 years. She lives alone but is visited regularly by her two daughters, who have grown-up families of their own. Over a period of two years, her daughters have noticed that Rose has become increasingly forgetful and they are becoming increasingly concerned for her welfare. Lately, Rose's short-term memory is very poor and she often forgets to eat or go shopping. Her appetite has always been poor, but she now has some signs of being underweight.

One of Rose's daughters lives in the same town and visits her several times a week. Rose's other daughter lives a two-hour drive away, but still visits regularly. However, on the last three occasions that she has arranged to visit her mother, she arrived to find that Rose had forgotten that her daughter was visiting and had gone out. Rose has been assessed by a psychiatrist and has a diagnosis of vascular dementia, which has been confirmed by an MRI scan.

Dementia is a condition in which there is a gradual loss of brain function with a concurrent decline in cognitive and intellectual ability. The main symptoms are usually loss of memory, confusion, problems with speech and understanding, changes in personality and behaviour and an increased reliance on others for help with the activities of daily living. It is not a disease in itself, but rather a group of symptoms that may result from age, brain injury, disease, vitamin deficiency, hormonal imbalance, misuse of drugs or excessive use of alcohol. A person with dementia may exhibit changes in mood, personality or behaviour. Confusion and disorientation may also be present. A diagnosis of dementia requires a loss of mental function severe enough to interfere with the patient's daily living.

Nevertheless, Rose still drives her car. Her daughters are worried as she has become lost on two recent occasions during the course of short local journeys. Patients who have a diagnosis of dementia are required by law to inform the Driver and Vehicle Licensing Authority (DVLA). In addition, it is possible that the motor insurance held by a person with dementia is likely to be invalidated if they do not declare their diagnosis to their insurance company. It seems ironic that current UK legislation requires a person with severe memory problems to remember to contact a government agency to inform them of their own condition. In reality, this situation frequently results in friction between the affected person and their carers in that the information may well have to be provided by the latter, possibly without the patient's consent, for the protection of the public. Health professionals are frequently approached to provide corroborating evidence in such circumstances.

Podiatric presentation

Rose has a hallux valgus deformity on her right foot. The degree of distortion is such that she finds it difficult to buy shoes that are wide enough to accommodate the prominent hallux valgus joint. In addition, she has very small feet, which were narrow prior to developing the hallux valgus. The position of the right hallux is now so acute that it sits on top of the second toe. This has resulted in her developing a large soft corn between these two digits, which is quite macerated as a result of a build up of sweat. Just recently, this corn has ulcerated owing to the excessive moisture within the tissues and has required podiatric intervention.

Challenge 1: How can the podiatrist reduce the number of missed appointments and enable Rose to be more concordant?

It is highly likely that Rose may forget her podiatric appointments, or attend at the wrong times. It is very helpful to patients with memory problems to be contacted prior to their appointment. However, it is important to seek the patient's permission to do so as some patients may be offended by an action that they believe to be unnecessary. Similarly, concordance with antibiotic treatment may be problematic for Rose. Antibiotics need to be taken regularly and the course completed in order for the treatment to be effective. Moreover, taking incomplete courses of antibiotics may increase the risk of developing antibiotic-resistant strains of bacteria. It may be helpful to Rose to be provided with a daily pill box with each dose labelled individually.

Challenge 2: What are the clinical and management challenges that Rose presents to the podiatrist?

Rose may not understand that the infected corn that she presents requires regular changes in dressings using an aseptic technique which needs to be undertaken by the podiatrist. In similar situations, Rose has often removed her dressings because she finds them irritating. However, she fails to appreciate the necessity for the dressings to be replaced and believes that allowing fresh air to be in contact with her wound is more beneficial than keeping it covered. At her latest visit to the podiatrist, the dressing appears to have been removed and replaced inappropriately. This provides a challenging clinical situation for the podiatrist to manage. On the one hand, patients such as Rose are vulnerable and require care and empathetic handling. On the other hand, people with dementia can be very frustrating to work with, because of the nature of their symptoms. For example, people who suffer short-term memory loss frequently repeat conversations, are unable to recall instructions and become confused easily. Even the most patient of practitioners may well find these characteristics frustrating, particularly in the context of a busy clinical practice, with the attendant time limitations common to contemporary practice. This potential difficulty may be best minimised by both an understanding of the needs of patients with dementia and the nature of the disease, together with a mindfulness of one's own reactions to such clients.

Dementia is an increasingly prevalent problem in Western society and is associated with an increasingly aged population. The prevalence in dementia increases with advancing years. Of people aged 40–64, approximately one per 1000 will suffer from dementia. Between the ages of 65 and 70, this figure rises sharply to one in 50 and still further for people aged 70 to 80, where one in 20 people are likely to have this condition. For people aged over 80 years, about one in five are likely to suffer from dementia. In total, it is estimated that in excess of 700 000 people in the United Kingdom have dementia at any given moment in time.

It is expected that this figure will rise to around 840 000 by 2010 and 1.5 million by 2050. Overall, this amounts to one person in every 120. Given that the mean age of patients attending for podiatry treatment tends to be greater than that of the wider population, the number of people seen in podiatric practice who have dementia is considerable. A number of forms of dementia exist. Around 55% of suffers have Alzheimer's disease, whilst a further 20% of people with symptoms of dementia will have vascular dementia. The remaining 25% of people presenting with dementia suffer from diseases affecting the Lewy bodies and the frontotemporal lobes of the brain (MedicineNet.com, 2009).

Despite its prevalence, dementia is a condition which has attracted both prejudice and ridicule. As a result, sufferers are likely to attempt to conceal their condition and be unwilling to seek help. In addition, dementia affects not only older people but is also increasingly recognised in middle-aged individuals. Although a higher profile for the disease has been sought by patients' advocates, dementia remains little understood by the public and is often treated dismissively.

Dementia is often progressive. Whilst it starts with increased lapses of short-term memory, during the latter stages of the disease personality changes may occur, which can be extremely distressing for relatives and friends of the sufferer. Many carers' state that the person is not the person they once knew. They experience a sense of loss, which has been likened to that of bereavement; in addition, carers bear the burden of looking after a loved one who may be demanding or unresponsive.

Because Rose forgets to eat regularly and may well keep inadequate food supplies in her home, her poor skin condition may be a result of her nutritional state particularly in relation to Vitamin B12 deficiencies. The prescription of B12 supplements may well be helpful in improving Rose's condition.

One of the most important considerations when working with people with dementia is the effect that the disease has upon their relatives and friends. It is extraordinarily distressing for partners or the children of a person with dementia to witness their slow but inexorable decline in mental capacity. Frequently, the individual's personality is affected, and a formerly affectionate mother or father may become argumentative or even aggressive. Conversely, it is not unknown for individuals who prior to the onset of disease were difficult to become more amiable. This brings its own set of difficulties for relatives who often experience feelings of guilt because of their earlier inability to engage with their relative's previously less-affable behaviour. The responsibility of caring for a relative with dementia can be very onerous, and many carers experience burnout as a result. When this occurs, carers frequently feel resentment towards the patient and subsequently experience feelings of guilt because of this.

Moreover, many carers of people with dementia are older people themselves. Frequently, the primary carer is the husband/wife/partner of the person affected. In the case of older patients, the children of the affected person may well be past retirement age themselves.

It is essential that the podiatrist is able to demonstrate empathetic responses towards the carers of patients with dementia who present for treatment. The podiatrist must be prepared to give time to listen carefully to their concerns and needs to be prepared to handle their frustrations and resentment sensitively and with skill.

Summary of important health psychology

The main feature for Rose is her dementia. Other factors to be considered include the expected physical changes associated with ageing, which may include loss of mobility and its consequent effects on psychological health, for example isolation. In this case, however, currently Rose is still able to drive her car, but this is a situation that cannot continue, and Rose's isolation will increase when she gives up driving. Those with dementia are often poorly nourished and dehydrated, resulting in an exacerbation of the symptoms of dementia.

The second major factor in Rose's care is her social isolation. Social isolation is an increasing problem in British society. In the United Kingdom, about one in six people is over the age of 65. Similarly, the number of older people living alone has risen and continues to rise. At the same time, the importance of social networks specifically among older people is beginning to be more widely recognised (Delisle, 1998). Such issues are particularly salient in the South-East of England, which contains both some of the most affluent and most deprived areas in the country in close geographical proximity.

Since Townsend (1962) first described the concept of *community care*, later empirical research has shown that most older people requiring care are looked after by partners or immediate family members, who are usually female (Qureshi and Walker, 1989). Subsequently, Wenger (1994) has made a major research contribution in this area. She suggests that a typology of support networks can be derived from the following factors:

- geographical proximity of close family
- the relative proportions of family, friends and neighbours involved in caring for the older person
- the older person's level of interaction with their family, friends, neighbours and groups in their community.

Wenger identifies five types of network:

1. **The family-dependent support network:** Older persons in this network type are generally over 80 years of age and are often widowed. The network is generally small, containing between one and four people, and

is characterised by interaction primarily with family, together with a few friends and/or neighbours. It may involve the older person sharing a household with adult children, or with their own siblings. Alternatively, they may live very near to such kin but in separate households.

2. **The locally integrated support network:** Individuals in this type of network are usually under 80 years of age and have lived in the same community since they were less than 40 years of age. They have frequent contact with their neighbours, and enjoy close relationships with their family, friends and neighbours. Such people often participate in their community, and their networks are large, including eight or more people.

3. **The local self-contained support network:** This type of network involves infrequent contact with at least one relative, but support is more usually focused on neighbours. However, contact is made only when it is felt necessary. Older people in this type of network generally participate in their local communities only to a very limited extent.

4. **The wider community focused support network:** This type of network is found largely among middle-class people living with a spouse. They are often retirement migrants, and may be 50 miles or more from their nearest child or sibling. Nonetheless, they maintain active relationships with distant relatives and with friends and a few neighbours. Geographical proximity is less important to such individuals than are friendship groups.

5. **Private restricted support network:** This type of network is characteristic of couples who moved to a locality after the age of 40. They have no local family and are often childless, or their nearest child lives more than 50 miles away.

Wenger and Shahtahmasebi (1990) and Wenger (1994) demonstrate that people in locally integrated support (type 2) networks tend to place the least, and people in private restricted support (type 5) networks the most, demands on health and social services, including social workers, community nurses, home helps, meals-on-wheels services and members of the clergy. Those in family-dependent support (type 1) networks also receive proportionately higher levels of visits from social workers, community nurses and the clergy, but utilise meals-on-wheels services and home helps less. Older people in local self-contained support (type 3) networks receive higher levels of visits from social workers, community nurses, home helps and the clergy, but only at advanced ages (over 80). People in locally integrated support (type 2) networks receive a higher level of visits only from the clergy. Successful interventions would therefore encourage movement from other types to locally integrated support networks, that is increasing the number and diversity of support networks. Such initiatives would both improve the quality of life for many older people and reduce the burden on statutory services. The potential of community development to inform the work of Primary Care groups has also been recognised (Fisher *et al.*, 1999).

Implications for podiatric management

The implications are twofold in that the direct podiatric foot management is straightforward. First, Rose requires adequate footwear, minute debridement of the painful corn, astringent treatment for the maceration and laboratory confirmation of any possible mycotic infection. Second, and of greater difficulty, is the maintenance of overall continuity of treatment. Very often, people with dementia fail to keep appointments, necessitating the need for reminders and prompts. It may become necessary in order to ensure contact with Rose that she is transferred to a domiciliary caseload and that she is seen at home. The advantage of this is that Rose will be more familiar with her own surroundings and her dementia may not be so problematic.

Recommended self-treatment at home is often neglected simply because the patient forgets and medication is often inappropriately taken for medical conditions.

Should Rose receive domiciliary treatment, the podiatrist should consider the environment in which she resides and act as part of the falls prevention team by identifying risks and hazards within the home. Trailing cables, curled mats and dim lighting are all potential hazards; of great significance are 'sloppy slippers'. Some local authority social services departments have a slipper exchange programme where inappropriate slippers are replaced free of charge. Early indications are that this scheme is contributing to the reduction in falls in older people. Where no such scheme exists, the podiatrist should make recommendations for appropriate slippers.

Chapter 16

Professional boundaries

If I talk, everyone thinks I'm showing off; when I'm silent, they think I'm ridiculous; rude if I answer, sly if I get a good idea, lazy if I'm tired, selfish if I eat a mouthful more than I should, stupid, cowardly, crafty, etc.

Anne Frank

Harriet Edmondson portrays many of the characteristics of adolescence. This chapter explores some of the difficulties the podiatrist may face when treating a young adult. Issues of professional boundaries are considered.

Harriet is a 15-year-old who is referred to your practice with an in-growing toenail. She is tall and slim and is wearing loose sportswear, consisting of tracksuit bottoms and an overlarge sweatshirt. Harriet has a thin face with high cheek bones, which are accentuated by her long hair being swept back tightly into a pony tail, which makes Harriet look rather severe. You have just completed an evening class in personal counselling and as a result have become quite observant of your patients' non-verbal behaviour. You notice that Harriet is a reserved girl with a sullen facial expression, which does not change when she engages in conversation. She avoids making eye contact with anyone, appears to be reticent and withdrawn and rather intense. Harriet reports that her in-growing toenail occurred as a result of a netball accident in which her opponent accidentally jumped and landed on her toe. Initially, the toe was inflamed and the nail was torn and ragged. Harriet reports that 'it felt like it had something sticking in it' and so she tried to 'tidy up' the nail with her nail scissors. Harriet reports that she plays netball twice a week at school and is a member of a local team. When she is not playing netball, she likes to keep fit by using the gym at her mother's fitness club.

Harriet is accompanied by her mother, who is extremely smart and wearing a well-cut business suit with expensive jewellery. She has an air of efficiency but a rather patronising conversational style. She is clearly irritated by her daughter's action to self-treat, which has resulted in this injury. She has been forced to take time off work to bring her daughter to the clinic for professional help. Conversation between Harriet and her mother is limited.

Podiatric presentation

Harriet is reluctant to let the podiatrist inspect her toe and is adamant that no one may touch it. Having been coaxed into removing her trainer and sock, she presents a toenail that is extremely red, swollen and oozing thick yellow pus. The sides of the toe are bulging and have exuded over the nail plate, leaving only a small amount of nail plate exposed. While she is indicating the point where the nail seems to be digging in, you notice that she has very bitten finger nails, and the skin around the nails has been picked, leaving the tissue raw and inflamed. Picking at finger and toenails is termed *onychotillomania*.

Factors influencing Harriet's behaviour

Harriet likes competition and competing; she says it makes her feel good and gives her a 'buzz'. She is a serious athlete and maintenance of fitness and her figure are extremely important to her. For a girl of 15 her face and overall physique appear to be extremely thin. However, it is difficult to assess this fully because the type of clothing she has chosen to wear covers her arms and legs completely. She seems nervous and picks at her fingers when not engaged in conversation.

Adolescence is the stage that represents the transition between childhood and adulthood, and an understanding of adolescent behaviour is important. Adolescence is a phase marked by significant physical changes including altered body shape. In addition, body image becomes more important, cognitive development accelerates and relations with adults, parents and authority may become difficult. It is a time of uncertainty, when decisions are made in relation to future careers and developments.

Marcia (1966) proposes the notion of an adolescent identity crisis, or a time when adolescents have no sense of a personal identity, which is characterised by strong feelings of uncertainty. Marcia suggests that adolescents tend to move from low identity status to high identity status as a result of growing external and internal pressures on them to enter the adult world. Erikson (1968) identifies stages in adolescent development and suggests that adolescence is a time when individuals strive to avoid role confusion.

In moving closer to adulthood, teenagers reach a point where they want to be defined by anything other than their parents. They want to stop spending so much time with their family, require independence and may distance themselves from their parents. The process of separation from parents is a gradual and natural one. Erik Erikson was the first psychologist to develop the notion of an adolescent *identity crisis*. He proposed that all of the earlier crystallisations of identity formed during childhood come into question during adolescence. Moreover, they coincide with the overwhelming combination of physical changes, increased sex drive, expanded mental abilities and increasing and conflicting social demands made upon young people. In order to develop a sense of identity amidst such confusion, Erikson (1968) suggests that adolescents need to try out a variety of roles and 'must often test extremes before settling on a considered course'.

It is also common for adolescents to reject their parents, and all that they stand for, in order that they can make a clean break from childhood in an attempt to create their identity. They often seek role models and can be rather indiscriminate about where they find them. Commonly, they will turn to peer groups to find the missing sense of belonging. Such behaviours help to explain some of the cult-like tendencies exhibited amongst early adolescents, who may worship the same heroes (movie stars, singers), wear the same clothes and 'rebel' against traditional authority. The interesting thing about this so-called rebellion is that it's often actually another form of conformity and an attempt to be accepted.

Role models can be highly influential and make a critical difference to the choices that adolescents make, choices that could affect the rest of their lives. Teenagers demonstrate a strong need to idealise others, especially those who are older and more worldly, and aspire to qualities that they desperately want to possess.

Adolescents therefore use peer groups to develop a sense of social identity. Waterman (1982) notes that adolescents who have affectionate parents who give them sufficient freedom to become individuals in their own right tend to have explored and considered different alternatives for themselves. By contrast, adolescents whose parents are domineering are less likely to have considered their own identity, while adolescents whose parents are aloof and uninvolved tended neither to have considered their identity nor to have any commitment to the future (Waterman, 1982).

While Harriet exhibits many typical features of adolescence, she also shows signs which would lead the podiatrist to suspect that all is not well.

Peer pressure is acknowledged to be highly influential during the adolescent period. At adolescence, peer relations expand to occupy a particularly central role in young people's lives. New types (for example opposite sex, romantic ties) and levels (for example crowds) of peer relationships emerge.

Peers typically replace the family as the centre of a young person's social and leisure activities. Teenagers have multiple peer relationships, and they confront multiple peer cultures that have remarkably different norms and value systems.

Peers can have extremely powerful influence in the teenage years. Estimates suggest that around one in six adolescents are bullied. Teenagers may be bullied by their peers for a number of reasons, including:

- appearance, such as being overweight
- resisting the pressure to conform
- background, including race and socio-economic factors
- academic achievement.

It is therefore important that vulnerable adolescents be provided with appropriate support in order to cope with such difficulties. Research suggests that friendships are very important to young people's overall growth, stability and personal development. Friends provide social and cognitive skills for each other that would otherwise be lacking. Having friends has proven to show positive outcomes in both boys and girls, and across different cultural groups, and different intelligence levels (Hartup, 1996).

Behavioural characteristics, attitudes and qualitative features of these relationships are all important factors in predicting the developmental outcomes of friendships (Hartup, 1996). While peer influence is neither good nor bad as a whole, it can go either way very easily based on the adolescents and the group as well as the dynamics that take place within the group.

Pre-adolescent children spend far less time with their friends and more time being monitored by adults, often their parents. Less time with other children, and more parental direction, makes for less peer influence. By contrast, adolescents seek less time with adults and more with peers. In the process of forming an independent identity, adolescents are relatively easily influenced as they seek their independence.

In general, most adolescents tend to follow similar paths to their independence. However, the presence of a few poorly adjusted individuals may have a profound influence on group behaviour. Pearson and Michell (2000) describe a process of *deviancy training* within some adolescent friendships, which results in increases in delinquency, substance use, violence and adult maladjustment.

The adolescent period is also a time when anorexia nervosa can develop. Anorexia nervosa is an eating disorder, which is thought to develop as a coping mechanism to both external and internal influences and conflicts.

People with anorexia usually have a perception of being overweight, and have a heightened sensitivity and fear of becoming fat. Anorexia nervosa is often associated with low self-esteem and the need for acceptance. It occurs primarily in adolescent females (12–25 years), and more commonly in families from higher socio-economic groups. Anorexia nervosa is 20 times more prevalent among females than males. Among ballet dancers, the prevalence may be as high as 3.5–7.6% (Nelson, 1996).

The most common features of anorexia nervosa are loss of weight, coupled with changes in behaviour. The weight loss is slowly progressive and often follows on from a weight-reducing diet. It is only after several months that it becomes clear that the dieting is pathological and the weight loss extreme. Initially, weight loss may be positively reinforced by favourable comments by friends and family about the individual's new, slimmer appearance. However, as the weight loss continues, attempts to challenge the sufferer's further dieting are usually met with anger, deceit or a combination of both. Often, families are ill equipped to deal with this situation and may resort to confrontation, bullying or bribery, all of which usually fail.

Increasing introversion is manifested by the sufferer, who becomes less outgoing, less sociable and less fun. Contact with friends may be lost and a lack of interest in everything apart from the avoidance of food and an increased commitment to academic work often become apparent. The person with anorexia may also display obsessive behaviour, especially in relation to food and exercise. This may be observed in the fastidious weighing of food, drinking abnormally large volumes of water and a marked increase in the intensity and duration of exercise. Excessive exercise is frequently observed in people with anorexia nervosa and has been considered to be both an addiction and an obsessive-compulsive disorder under these circumstances (Davis et al., 1999). Loss of confidence and assertiveness are often seen in people suffering from anorexia, who may become less argumentative and more dependent on others. At the same time, their anorexic behaviour will increasingly control the lives of those close to them.

The causes of anorexia nervosa appear to be multifactorial. Factors may include personality, aspects of family members and relationships within the family. External stresses and problems with friendships at school are often factors in the aetiology. The increased incidence of anorexia nervosa in families where there are other anorexics may indicate a genetic predisposition.

People predisposed to anorexia tend to be conformist, compliant and hard working. They are often popular with teachers and may appear to given little cause for worry over the years. As their contemporaries go through the difficulties of adolescence, they seem models of sensible behaviour by comparison. These traits may be quite marked before the onset of anorexia but they are usually accentuated by the disorder.

Osteoporosis and amenorrhea are symptoms of a hormonal imbalance brought about by anorexia nervosa (Nishizawa *et al.*, 2001). This is because the disorder not only interrupts the normal rapid bone accretion charac-teristics of adolescents but also accelerates bone loss. Low body mass and low calcium intake contribute further to the risk of osteoporosis.

Harriet may see the podiatrist as an establishment figure, which could create difficulties in establishing a relationship. Paton and Brown (1991) suggest that health professionals communicating with adolescents require a sensitive approach in order that they are not perceived as a 'parent'. Often, discussions of a personal nature are particularly embarrassing for adolescents, and they may be reluctant to reveal their anxieties for fear of being considered 'silly'. All adolescents feel particularly self-conscious about their bodies, and podiatrists need to ensure adolescent patients feel confident that their privacy and confidentiality are guaranteed.

Challenge 1: Should you broach the subject of Harriet's suspected anorexia nervosa?

You suspect that Harriet may be suffering from anorexia nervosa. You have attended a part-time counselling course in which eating disorders were discussed. Is Harriet's suspected condition an issue that you should address?

Anorexia nervosa is a condition whose aetiology is complex and not always well understood. Its treatment is difficult and not always successful. It is very unlikely that the podiatrist will have the experience, skills or time necessary to intervene in Harriet's case and it is important that podiatrists are cognisant of the limits of their professional competence. However, it may be very difficult for the podiatrist to ignore the natural desire to help. If this is the case, then any approach should be made confidentially through Harriet's mother, as Harriet is likely to be defensive of her eating behaviour. This is complicated in Harriet's case, as her relationship with her mother appears to be strained. It should also be noted that Harriet is below the age of consent for medical treatment should any referral be considered.

The presentation of the toenail indicates that Harriet may need a minor surgical procedure. As the nail is so painful, this will require the careful administration of an injection of local anaesthetic to block the pain sensation.

Consider how you will deliver this information to Harriet.

Challenge 2: What psychological issues will you consider prior to performing any surgical procedure?

Chapman and Kishore (1999) report on pre-operative anxiety and patients' information needs, and the findings are consistent with the much larger nursing literature in which the physical and psychological needs of patients undergoing elective day surgery (Mitchell, 1997; Calvin and Lane, 1999), and in particular the needs of children experiencing day surgery (Murphy-Taylor, 1999), are considered.

Miller (1980) suggests that patients awaiting surgery may act in one of two ways with regard to their desire for information. Those she calls *monitors* seek out as much information as possible concerning their condition and its treatment in order to reduce their anxiety. By contrast, those Miller describes as *blunters* prefer not to know what is to happen to them, and avoid such information as much as possible. Patients who are monitors are thus likely to find the delivery of pre-operative information beneficial in reducing anxiety. However, patients who are blunters may find such information raises their anxiety.

It may be helpful for some patients undergoing minor surgery under local anaesthetic to be given some control over the procedure in order to reduce their anxiety. Taylor (1986) suggests that there are four kinds of control involved:

1. **Behavioural control** involves the patient being able to control the progress of a procedure in some way and this reduces anxiety, e.g. when the patient is given control by an agreement that the procedure will stop on a predetermined signal, such as raising a hand.
2. **Cognitive control** involves the use of distraction techniques to concentrate the patient's thoughts on things other than the procedure, e.g. the use of relaxing music.
3. **Decision control** involves the patient having some influence when they are ready and wish to have the procedure performed
4. And the effectiveness of **information control** is illustrated in the case of Miller's (1980) monitors, who find the provision of information reassuring.

Harriet's general health is a cause for concern. She is currently debilitated through malnutrition and her healing ability is likely to be compromised. Your management of this should thus include arranging the provision of antibiotic therapy from her GP. It will be necessary for you to obtain Harriet's and her mother's consent for you to approach Harriet's doctor to ensure there are no contraindications to the surgery.

The provision of information for post-operative care is important for patients undergoing nail surgery. For Harriet, this advice will involve her stopping her exercise routine temporarily. This is likely to be difficult for her and so telling Harriet will require skill and tact on the part of the podiatrist.

Summary of important health psychology

Adolescence is always a period characterised by emotional instability. Adolescents may be volatile in their relationships with adults in general, and their parents in particular. Adolescents searching for a sense of identity may respond to encouragement to look inside themselves, rather than outside, for the answers. However, this is not always easy and may need to be undertaken by a skilled counsellor.

Anorexia is an uncommon but potentially extremely serious condition, which requires specialist intervention. It is essential for health professionals to be aware of and work within the limitations of their own competence and scope of practice. It is also important for practitioners to restrict their practice to that of the context in which they are working.

Implications for podiatric management

As previously stated, Harriet may be anxious with regard to the local anaesthetic injection. The podiatrist must also consider the significance of the infection and how this will be managed. Finally, careful assessment of the healing wound must be made and monitored especially considering the suspicion that you have that Harriet picks at her toenails. The condition, if carefully managed, is completely curable.

Chapter 17

Homelessness and people with complex needs

My weariness amazes me, I'm branded on my feet,
I have no one to meet. And the ancient empty street's
too dead for dreaming . . .

Bob Dylan

John Piper is a 42-year-old man who became homeless following the breakdown of his marriage and the death of his son. Subsequently, he spent some time in prison, from where he was released two years ago. The local authority's position regarding the housing of ex-offenders was such that they were unable to offer him any temporary accommodation. This, they explained, was because they considered him to have made himself homeless as a result of his conviction and subsequent prison sentence. However, this may not have been the case for other local authorities, who might have been able to offer John some housing support. Following his release, John was housed in temporary accommodation provided by a charitable organisation. However, his unacceptably disruptive behaviour led to his eviction, which resulted in him living on the streets. He has been in this situation intermittently ever since. Currently, John is on the housing waiting list, but there are several people ahead of him.

John's medical history includes epilepsy, which is controlled by medication, but he has a tendency to lose his prescriptions and to fail to attend appointments with his GP. John has a long-standing history of alcohol abuse, which has contributed to him being unable to secure accommodation. John has recently attended an interview at Golding House, a local sheltered accommodation provision for homeless people, but the staff there are reluctant to offer him a place because of his unwillingness to address his alcohol dependency.

Five days ago, John fell from a high ledge whilst intoxicated. He was admitted to the local Emergency Department and underwent an internal fixation procedure for a fractured tibia and fibula. John refused to stay in hospital following his surgery, and discharged himself within a few hours of his operation. He later revealed that he did not trust hospitals because it was in hospital that his son had died.

John attends the day centre and health centre run by local voluntary services. They offer showers, clean clothing, hot food, together with podiatric and nursing care. The podiatrist's role includes offering foot treatment and foot health advice. There are a number of specific foot conditions associated with homelessness, which include poor footwear, poor foot hygiene, infestation, together with the effects of cold and prolonged wet conditions, including trench foot and frost bite.

Podiatric presentation

John presented at the clinic with an infected surgical wound that was malodorous and oozing, and had associated ascending cellulitis above the ankle joint. He was also in considerable pain.

The podiatrist and nurse have treated the wound with dressings and antibiotics. Despite having been prescribed several courses of antibiotics, there has been little marked improvement in John's wound. He admits that he has not always taken his antibiotics, claiming that they 'make him feel sick'. Additionally, John has not been eating properly and has lost weight. He often goes for a couple of days without food and is once again sleeping on the streets. In addition to this, he is well known to the local police.

John had not attended the day centre for a week. Staff were concerned and had spoken with some of the other regular clients to see if any of them knew of his whereabouts. One client reported that John had been admitted to hospital a few days previously. Staff at the hospital reported that John had experienced an epileptic fit. His leg was also found to have developed osteomyelitis. Whilst in hospital, John was treated with intravenous antibiotics and underwent surgery to remove the internal fixation devices. In order to obtain some accommodation for John, a hospital doctor faxed a referral to the housing unit, stressing that his need for accommodation was urgent. However, John failed to attend for the housing interview and contact with him was lost at this point.

A few weeks later, at the beginning of the Bank Holiday weekend, John arrived at the day centre 10 minutes before closing time. He was very drunk and was demanding that accommodation be found for him for that night. Staff tried to explain that there was no emergency accommodation available at any of their units. They also explained that the units would not accept him in his present state as they have strict rules about the use of alcohol by their residents. John swore at the staff and denied that he was drunk, before storming out.

Subsequently, he has come into the clinic irregularly to have his wound redressed. The wound does appear smaller and less infected. However, John is due to be admitted to hospital in a few days' time, as there are still concerns that the bones are infected. If this is the case, he will need a further operation and will need to spend four to six weeks in hospital.

The podiatrist at Golding House has been seeing John occasionally, offering advice regarding how to protect his feet whilst living on the streets and concerning his general foot health care.

Factors influencing John's behaviour

Chaotic lifestyles are often seen in people with substance misuse problems, and such individuals can often become disengaged from services. Benjaminsen et al. (1990) conducted a study to investigate factors relating to suicidal behaviour amongst people with alcohol problems. This study showed that over a third of the subjects had attempted suicide at least once. Attempters were more likely to have suffered from depression, feelings of hopelessness, anxiety attacks, agoraphobia and to have misused substances. In regard to coping strategies, attempters were less likely to make plans or to make the best of a stressful situation by attempting to learn from it. They were more likely to disengage, to resort to denial or to alcohol or drugs when faced with stressful events than were subjects who had not attempted suicide.

John's reasons for drinking may be deep-rooted and may prove difficult to change. John had revealed to staff that his son had died in hospital and that this caused his drinking to become uncontrolled. John's drinking had also increased whilst living on the streets.

If John were found suitable housing, he might be able to reduce his alcohol intake. Because of the length of time that John has misused alcohol and because of the reasons for his alcohol use, total abstinence is likely to be an unrealistic aim. It may be helpful to involve local alcohol services at this point, including those services available in the voluntary sector.

Housing is also an important factor in John's management. The increased risk of mortality in the homeless population is well documented. Cheung and Hwang (2004) found that homeless women aged 18 to 44 were 10 times more likely to die than were women of a similar age in the general population. Mortality rates were also found to be elevated amongst the male homeless population. Barrow et al. (1999) found that homeless men were four times more likely to die than were men of a similar age in the general population. The likelihood of mortality amongst homeless men is increased by chronic homelessness, substance misuse and prior imprisonment. In contrast to the general population, the mean age of death for homeless people is thought to be 44.5 years (Ishorst-Witte *et al.*, 2001).

Challenge 1: Identifying support mechanisms

Finding solutions to John's difficulties associated with alcohol misuse and housing may prove difficult. Nevertheless, health professionals working in this field are in a unique position to provide support to John and to act as an advocate for him when engaging with statutory organisations, such as local authority services. Keeping John in contact with people in the voluntary sector alone is better than complete disengagement, which leaves John more at risk.

Challenge 2: Strategies for dealing with substance misuse

There are several things that we can do as health professionals to support people in John's situation:

- **Listening and accepting the situation**: it is important to gain his trust and emphasise our respect for his confidentiality.
- **Social support** plays a key part in John's treatment plan. Patients who have some form of social support are much more likely to allow the intervention of health services.
- **Advocacy**: speaking on the behalf of others who don't have a voice. Advocacy assists people in engaging with other services and in making them aware of people's needs.
- **Being flexible**: being flexible to John's needs may include being open to negotiation about appointment times, and accompanying John to other appointments and meetings with service providers.
- **Recognising stages of readiness to change**: is John contemplating change or not considering it at all? The Stages of Change Model is discussed in more detail in Chapter 21.
- **Approaching one problem at a time**: people in John's situation have many problems that may include substance misuse, smoking, housing issues and physical and/or mental health issues. By concentrating on the most important problem first, you are more likely to retain engagement.
- **Communicating clearly** is essential. This may include the use of street language and an appreciation of the effects of the drugs people use and the amounts that they regularly consume. Such discussions may

be initially uncomfortable for inexperienced professionals but practice improves confidence.

- **Making the most of every contact**: because the chaotic lifestyle of homeless people may provide limited opportunities to help. Conversely, there are a number of things which are less helpful when working with people like John.
- **Rescuing**: it may be tempting to try and 'rescue' the person and take control of their lives. Although advocacy is important, there must also be an emphasis on encouraging self-confidence and empowering the patient to act for themselves.
- **Assuming that the patient has the same inner resources and control to make decisions that the professional has**: because of their situation, many homeless people lack the internal locus of control necessary to initiate change.
- **Being judgemental**: this will lead to disengagement and will render you unapproachable.

In dealing with people with multiple needs, it is important to establish realistic treatment plans that are amenable to the patient. It is also important to recognise that these patients may put needs such as warmth, shelter and food above your priorities. It can be easy to assume that such patients will conform to 'normal' patient behaviours, such as attending appointments, changing dressings and home treatments. As practitioners, it is important to widen our view of what is normal. Patients with multiple needs need particular support, and this may include tasks that are outside our normal areas of practice. For example, accompanying patients to other appointments may not be seen as a routine part of the podiatrist's role. Nevertheless, it may make the difference between a successful and an unsuccessful outcome.

Summary of important health psychology

When working with patients with multiple needs, it is essential to be flexible in our approach to notions of normality, professional roles and the care that we provide. Sometimes, professional divisions need to be set aside in order to gain the best outcome for our patients. Although this may be difficult in some settings, it is possible in the voluntary sector and should be encouraged in the statutory sector wherever possible.

Implications for podiatric management

Working in the multidisciplinary team is the cornerstone of satisfactory podiatric management for all patients. This is particularly the case when dealing with the complex needs of homeless people. Without close collaboration of all those involved in John's care, it is unlikely that his state of health will show any appreciable improvement. John's alcohol use, housing and nutritional state all impact on his tissue viability, and excluding his social needs from our treatment plans will not bring about an improvement in his podiatric condition.

Chapter 18

Social factors versus medical needs

The Family is the Country of the heart. There is an angel in the Family who, by the mysterious influence of grace, of sweetness, and of love, renders the fulfilment of duties less wearisome, sorrows less bitter.

Giuseppe Mazzini

Social factors are sometimes more significant to a patient than are their medical needs. Understanding the motivations and values of a patient is necessary in order to understand and explain their behaviours.

Margaret Knowles is a 60-year-old woman who lives in a one-bedroom flat on the sixteenth floor of a tower block. The block of flats was built in the 1960s and has a dreary appearance, being constructed from concrete. The area demonstrates little architectural attractiveness. The ground floor is defaced by graffiti and the lift is regularly out of order. The few shops nearby which are still trading have metal shuttering, erected at night to prevent vandalism. The local community has few facilities and has neither a health nor community centre. Unemployment rates are above average, and the older local residents are fearful of being out after dark.

Margaret lives alone, having been widowed 15 years ago. She has a daughter, who is a lone parent, who lives in a nearby block of flats with her two children. Margaret helps to look after her grandchildren, enabling her daughter to work part-time and to have an occasional break from childcare. Margaret works as a shelf stacker at the local convenience store. She likes the flexibility of the work, which enables her to pick up her grandchildren after school each day. Every fourth week, she takes the opportunity of visiting the podiatrist, whose surgery is in the centre of town and close by her grandchildren's school. The children attend a Roman Catholic School, which is located approximately 10 minutes' walk from the podiatrist's surgery. Margaret enjoys spending time with her grandchildren, who bring joy and pleasure into her otherwise dull life.

Podiatric presentation

Margaret has rigid highly arched feet with deep seated painful corns over the metatarsal heads. Podiatry treatment is required every three to four weeks to keep her pain-free and able to walk comfortably.

She has been a patient in the practice for over three years and has developed a friendly and comfortable relationship with the podiatrist. Over a period of two to three months, the podiatrist has noticed that Margaret is becoming distant and appears very tired. On some occasions, conversation between them has become uncharacteristically stilted and the podiatrist has noticed that she is becoming evasive. At about this time, the podiatrist also notices that Margaret is using an increasing amount of perfume. As the weeks pass, this has become more obvious until the podiatrist feels obliged to comment. It is at this point that Margaret finally broke down and revealed that she had been very worried about her health for some months.

She said, 'Would you mind if I showed you what's been troubling me? It's got nothing to do with my feet, but I don't know who else to turn to.'

Margaret unbuttoned her blouse, removed layers of bandages and padding from her breast, finally revealing what was obviously a fungating tumour. The wound was deep with a purulent offensive discharge. It was at this point that she started to cry.

She explained that she was terrified to go to her doctor for a number of reasons. She was fearful of a diagnosis of cancer, believing that this is always fatal. She was concerned about letting her daughter and grandchildren down, worrying that the treatment would involve hospitalisation. In addition, a stay in hospital would mean that her daughter could not work. Margaret feared that she would not be able to help with the grandchildren, and that she would inevitably lose touch with them. She also believed that any treatment for cancer would inevitably necessitate prolonged aftercare and convalescence, which would result in her becoming a 'burden' to her daughter.

Illness behaviour and perceptions of illness are important concepts. The same 'illness' may be experienced differently by different people and have different meanings for them. This individual experience of illness results in people behaving in individual ways (Kasl and Cobb, 1966).

Furthermore, a patient's perception of symptoms may not correlate to the seriousness of the condition. Patients' perceptions of illness or disease severity may have a cultural component, and the manner in which an individual is meant to respond is culturally determined.

People from different cultural backgrounds report pain, and behave, in different ways, which are acceptable to, and expected in, their cultures. In a seminal piece of work conducted in a New York hospital, Zborowski (1952) reported that male Jewish patients tended to articulate their feelings with 'passion'. By contrast what Zborowski (1952) describes as 'old American' (Caucasian, non-Jewish) patients behaved with stoicism because emotional outbursts were viewed as embarrassing by their families. Italians and patients from Hispanic cultures behaved similarly, and when in pain demonstrated great emotional outbursts of sorrow and anger. Such behaviours were regarded as acceptable by Italian and Hispanic families.

A patient's perception of their illness is dependent upon their previous experience and knowledge of that condition. Symptoms do not always result in medical consultation. When people experience unusual, abnormal or persistent symptoms, they turn to what is known as the *lay referral system*. This system involves consulting family and friends for advice about their condition (Cameron *et al.*, 1995). More importantly, it is through the lay referral system that the patient learns how he/she is *meant* to respond to their symptoms – in a way which is normatively acceptable.

Seeking professional help may be further delayed as a result of fear, ignorance of the condition and because of embarrassment. The way in which patients describe their symptoms varies widely and is affected by cultural and demographic factors. Many people who experience symptoms choose to wait to see whether they develop further before seeking professional advice.

Disease is not always characterised by the presence of symptoms. Even when symptoms are present, the pattern of their presentation is not always consistent. The lay referral system also serves to interpret what may be confusing and unfamiliar experiences. Leventhal and Benyamini (1997) suggest that the relationship of symptoms and diagnosis is in some ways reciprocal: people who experience symptoms tend to seek a diagnosis, while people who are given a diagnosis tend to seek symptoms consistent with that diagnosis.

Not all people respond to symptoms in ways which appear logical. Reactions to symptoms and lay beliefs about illness may result in behaviours which can range from complete denial of the illness through to a preoccupation with somatic symptoms. It is the task of the podiatrist to tease out the health beliefs of patients in order to reach an understanding of the patient's illness perceptions. An understanding of the patient's perspective, and thus behaviour, enables the podiatrist to tailor support to meet the needs of the patient.

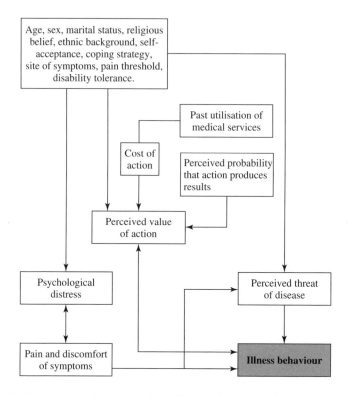

Figure 18.1 A structuralist approach to illness behaviour. (Adapted from Kasl and Cobb (1966), from Bond and Bond (1994))

There are various models which have been proposed to explain illness behaviour. Kasl and Cobb (1966) propose a structuralist approach (Figure 18.1). The structuralist approach suggests that people's behaviours, attitudes and values occur as a result of the organisation and structure of the society in which they live. The approach does not explain why people with similar social characteristics behave differently when experiencing similar symptoms.

As long ago as 1956, Beecher noted that individuals with injuries resulting in similar injury damage reacted differently. The manner in which the injury occurred determined the way in which the resultant damage was perceived. Injuries sustained by soldiers which resulted in the granting of home leave were evaluated differently from similar injuries suffered by factory workers that occurred in their workplace. Beecher (1956) suggests that for the soldiers the benefits resulting from the injury may compensate for the costs involved. In addition, soldiers injured during active service requested fewer doses of analgesia than did civilians injured in the workplace who suffered comparable injuries. This may explain why Margaret has been reluctant to seek advice regarding her breast tumour. Margaret's need to continue to assist her daughter and grandchildren is greater than her need to seek advice for her medical condition. The apparent illogicality of Margaret's behaviour is thus easily understood.

When patients become ill, they seek ways to explain and understand what has happened to them. It may be hard to make sense of what has happened, particularly if they have never experienced the symptoms or have been given a diagnosis. People often ask, 'Why me?' or 'Why now?' and seek explanations for their predicament based on considerations of personal history, lifestyle and behaviour.

For some people, symptoms must be taken seriously by *others* before the sufferer regards them as legitimate and can therefore define themselves as *being ill* (Senior and Viveash, 1998). People develop theories about their illness through consideration of their own experience, that of their families, friends and from knowledge gained from the media. Scharloo *et al.* (1998) suggest that there are five dimensions to the perceptions of illness:

- the problem, including signs, symptoms and labelling
- the cause of the problem
- the consequences of the problem
- the natural history and prognosis of the illness
- the cure/controllability of the illness.

Some or all of these dimensions are considered by the individual when making decisions about their health behaviour.

Heider (1958) proposes explanations for how people view their own behaviour and that of others. These explanations have become known as *attribution theory*. Attribution is said to be operationalised in two different ways. The first is known as *dispositional attribution*, in which a person's behaviour maybe explained by the presence of a stable characteristic, for example always being late. The second is known as *situational attribution*, in which a behaviour may be explained by external factors over which the individual has no personal control, for example being late as a result of traffic congestion.

In Margaret's case, it may be that dispositional and situational attributions might have combined to prevent her from seeking advice for her condition. On one hand, her disposition is such that she stoically refuses to 'make a fuss' about her own health. On the other hand, she has a daughter who is a lone parent who needs her help. Together, these factors may explain her behaviour.

In general, people's health status is influenced by their social, environmental and economic circumstances, in addition to their access to and uptake of medical services. People in higher socio-economic groups enjoy better health and enjoy lower morbidity and mortality rates than do those in lower socio-economic groups (Phillimore and Beattie, 1994).

Challenge 1: How can you deal with the powerful emotions elicited by Margaret's case?

When patients express powerful emotions, such as sadness, grief and anxiety, it may be difficult for the podiatrist not to share these feelings with their patients. In Margaret's case, how could you deal with such feelings whilst remaining helpful to her?

If you lack the skills to deal with your patient's emotions appropriately, you may feel inadequate and uncomfortable. Margaret's situation is such that it is unlikely that anyone would be prepared adequately for the emotional impact her case presents.

When a person is acutely upset, it is important not to attempt to prevent them from expressing emotion. It is helpful to find a private space away from others so that their distress is not further compounded by embarrassment.

When the patient has regained some composure, they should be allowed to articulate their concerns without pressure or interruption. Most importantly, the podiatrist should *listen* to what their patient is saying. Specialist counselling skills and qualifications are *not* required to be of real help and comfort to people who are acutely distressed. A warm and empathetic approach, and one expressing concern, will often prove very effective in making a distressed patient feel less so. After the patient has left the clinic, it is important for the podiatrist to reflect on how he/she has handled the situation and on how he/she may respond better in future. This process is often referred to as *reflective practice.*

Reflective practice

This is a means by which practitioners can develop a greater self-awareness about the nature and impact of their performance, an awareness that creates opportunities for professional growth and development (Osterman and Kottkamp, 1993). Maximum benefits from reflection are said to occur when the process happens in community, in interaction with others; when participants value the personal and intellectual growth of themselves and others; and when participants have time to engage in slow, non-assumptive thinking (Rogers, 2002).

■ Reflection is a meaning-making process, the thread that makes continuity of learning possible.

- Reflection is a systematic, rigorous, disciplined way of thinking, with its roots in scientific inquiry.
- Reflection needs to happen in community, in interaction with others.
- Reflection requires attitudes that value the personal and intellectual growth of oneself and of others.

What does reflective practice involve?

By developing and using reflective practice, the practitioner will be able to bring forward ideas to help improve and enhance practice and the practice of others. Effective practitioners continually reflect on their work and continue to do so throughout their careers.

The reflective process

The following six-stage process (Figure 18.2) is one example of a tool that may help to structure and gain the most benefit from your reflective analysis. By using these stages, it is possible to generate a series of questions which help structure the process of reflection to maximise the potential or actual changes in behaviour:

Reflective practice is a primary skill based on self-awareness. It links what we know, feel and think to what we observe in ourselves and in others. This

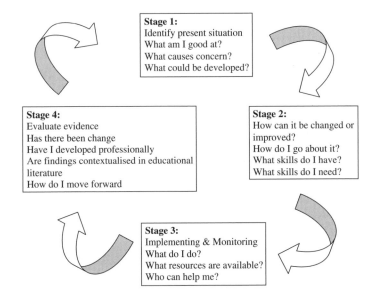

Stage 1:
Identify present situation
What am I good at?
What causes concern?
What could be developed?

Stage 4:
Evaluate evidence
Has there been change
Have I developed professionally
Are findings contextualised in educational literature
How do I move forward

Stage 2:
How can it be changed or improved?
How do I go about it?
What skills do I have?
What skills do I need?

Stage 3:
Implementing & Monitoring
What do I do?
What resources are available?
Who can help me?

Figure 18.2 The four stages of reflective practice

process helps to formalise how the practitioner sees their world, and how they organise and interpret information in professional practice. Where there is misunderstanding between the patient and the podiatrist, conflict and feelings of unease can occur. Reflective practice allows the podiatrist to learn from experience and to prevent the occurrence of similar problems in the future. It is thus very important for the podiatrist to reflect on how their reaction to patients' feelings influences their own feelings and actions.

Challenge 2: How can you moderate your own responses to unpleasant or frightening stimuli in order to avoid embarrassing your patient?

There will be times when the podiatrist will be presented with sights that may be alarming and smells that are far from pleasant. In such situations, it is important that the podiatrist maintain a professional and non-judgemental demeanour. It may be helpful to engage in general conversation to distract the patient from any non-verbal signals that you may be displaying inadvertently. It is also helpful to make regular eye contact and maintain a warm and friendly manner. When advice is being offered, particularly with regard to personal hygiene, a neutral and non-judgemental approach should be employed.

With experience, you will find that you react less acutely to unpleasant sights and smells. You will find that you are able to tolerate such situations without displaying signs of distaste. Inevitably, this results in a better and more comfortable experience for both you and the patient.

Summary of important health psychology

The social factors which determine Margaret's actions are more significant to her than are her medical needs. It is important for podiatrists to have a clear understanding of the motivations and values of their patients in order to act in a non-discriminatory or judgemental way. In order to achieve such understanding, podiatrists need to have an understanding of the basis of illness behaviour. Patients often behave in ways which may not appear to be logical to the podiatrist at first sight.

Implications for podiatric management

The treatment and management for Margaret's feet include skilled debridement of callus and corns and the use of appropriate keratolytics in conjunction with offloading orthotic devices. In order to accomplish this, suitable footwear is an absolute requirement. Extra-depth shoes should be sourced. Should improvements fail to be achieved in terms of pain and lesion reduction, electrocautery of the painful corns should be considered.

Postscript

Margaret commenced treatment for her breast tumour shortly after its discovery by the podiatrist. Unfortunately, her condition was too advanced to respond to surgery or therapy, and Margaret died a few months later.

Chapter 19

The importance of positivity

From quiet homes and first beginning,
Out to the undiscovered ends,
There's nothing worth the wear of winning,
But laughter and the love of friends.

Hilaire Belloc

The character of Dorothy Atkins is used to highlight the importance of positive traits and the positive effect that family and social ties can have on illness. Self-efficacy, control and optimism are each discussed in the context of this patient.

Dorothy is a 63-year-old married lady who has two grown-up children and four 'delightful' grandchildren. Dorothy and her husband have had a very happy life and have enjoyed her husband's retirement. They have lots of friends, have an active social life, being members of the local bowls club and horticultural society, and enjoy spending time with their family. Dorothy is a very happy person and feels that she has had a fulfilled and satisfying life.

Six months ago, Dorothy detected a small lump in her right breast, which was subsequently diagnosed as cancerous and resulted in Dorothy having a mastectomy and a course of chemotherapy. Dorothy has been optimistic throughout this period and believes that the treatment will return her to full health. She has been supported by her family and friends and has joined the local support group, which she has found most beneficial.

Podiatric presentation

Dorothy has attended the podiatrist recently for treatment of a fungal infection.

Factors influencing Dorothy's behaviour

Dorothy is a very positive, optimistic person who has derived much strength from her supportive family and from her network of friends.

Important psychological theory

Dorothy exhibits optimism and a high degree of self-efficacy. *Self-efficacy* is a characteristic which represents the degree of confidence a person has in their ability to perform certain behaviours. Self-efficacy has been shown to be associated with a variety of health outcomes (Grembowski *et al.*, 1993). *Optimism* is regarded as the quality of displaying favourable expectations for the future.

There is evidence to suggest that social support and ongoing membership of a social network are important in maintaining self-efficacy in later life. McAvay *et al.* (1996) found that a decline in health and self-efficacy were related to poorer social networks and fewer social contacts. There is also evidence of the reciprocal nature of the relationship between self-efficacy and social support: the impact of social support is to enhance self-efficacy and vice versa (Holahan and Holahan, 1987).

Dorothy also demonstrates a high degree of hardiness, which is related to self-efficacy and is characterised by a sense of personal control and commitment. Hardiness provides Dorothy with some of the emotional strength which helps her deal with her condition. She holds strong beliefs about the causes and consequences of her illness. These beliefs have been developed through her wide reading about cancer and cancer treatments.

Dorothy also believes strongly that she can influence the outcome of her illness. She shows a strong general motivation, a characteristic necessary to obtain positive outcomes (Dunn, 1996).

Locus of control is a concept which has been applied very widely in health psychology. The original theory was proposed by Rotter (1966) and has been the subject of much psychological research. People are said to have an *internal locus of control* if they believe that they have the ability to control events around them. By contrast, people are said to have an *external locus of control* if they believe that things that happen to them are largely controlled by outside influences. Levenson (1981) later suggested that the concept of locus of control was multidimensional. He proposed that external control had two components: the belief that events are random and controlled by chance and the belief that events are under the control of powerful others. Other authors have applied the concept to health-related behaviours. Wallstone and Wallstone (1978) developed the original Health Locus of Control scale. It is composed of Internal Health Locus of Control (IHLC), Powerful Others Health Locus of Control (PHLC) and Chance Health

Locus of Control (CHLC). Although medical practitioners were the subject of the 'Powerful Others Scale' in Wallstone and Wallstone's original work, it has been recognised more recently that a wider range of individuals may be substantially influential on an individual's behaviour.

It is important for the podiatrist to assess Dorothy's health knowledge and explore her health beliefs because these can influence her. This concept is explored in detail in Chapter 6. When in discussion with patients, it is important for practitioners to recognise that patients have access to a wide range of health-related information which will significantly influence their behavioural beliefs. It is also very important to be aware that a patient's friends and family play a pivotal role in their recovery.

Challenge 1: Explain why Dorothy is able to remain so cheerful despite having been diagnosed with a life-threatening condition

Many studies have demonstrated the independent effect of social networks on health status, morbidity and mortality rates. Perhaps the most important of these studies was the one conducted in Alameda County, California (Seeman *et al.*, 1987). Nearly 7000 adults were studied over a nine-year period. At the beginning of the period, subjects' social networks were recorded. Notes were taken of the subjects' number of relatives and friends, their membership of church and social groups and of the contact that the subject had with supportive others. Mortality and morbidity rates were then recorded in the same cohort nine years later. The study demonstrated clearly that those people with poorer social and community ties were far more likely to have died during the study period than were those who had better social networks. The age-adjusted relative risks for socially isolated people compared to those with the most social contacts were 2.3 for men and 2.8 for women. This effect was found to be independent of self-reported physical health status at the beginning of the study, year of death, socio-economic status and all major health behaviours, such as cigarette smoking, alcohol consumption, obesity, physical inactivity and use of health services. Similar findings have been reported in a prospective study of older men in Sweden (Hanson *et al.*, 1990). Five hundred men born in 1914 were interviewed and examined in 1982/3. A higher mortality risk was found for men with a lower availability of emotional support and who reported lower levels of social participation. This was particularly the case for men who lived alone. In these subjects, the relative risks for mortality were found to be in the range of 2.2 to 2.5 after adjustments for social class, health status at baseline, cardiovascular risk factors, alcohol intake, physical activity and body mass index had been made.

More recently, an 11-year longitudinal study of older men and women in Denmark showed a similar independent association between social relations and mortality risks. In this study, social relations were assessed by:

■ structural considerations, such as household composition, the presence of children and frequency of contact with relatives
■ the function of social relations, such as support with activities of daily living
■ participation in tasks which bring individuals together, such as volunteer work.

The study not only showed an association between social relations and mortality consistent with the American and Swedish studies but also demonstrated that two aspects of social relationships were particularly important. First, it is important for individuals to receive support with a range of everyday tasks. Second, it appears to be protective to help others, thus providing a sense of belonging and of usefulness to society.

In addition to improving quality of life and longevity, there is evidence to suggest that strong social networks may prevent or reduce disease processes, particularly in middle-aged and older people. A very large number ($n =$ in excess of 32 000) of male health professionals in the United States aged 42–77 entered a study in 1988 (Kawachi *et al.*, 1997). At the time, all participants were free from known coronary heart disease, stroke and cancer. Four years later, a total of 511 of the subjects had died. Socially isolated men (defined as unmarried, with fewer than six friends/relatives and with no membership of church or community groups) were found to be at increased risk of cardiovascular disease, accidents and suicide. Socially isolated men were also found to have a risk of stroke of more than twice that of men with the most extensive social networks. While the study found no evidence for the effects of social networking on non-fatal heart disease, it concluded that social networks assist in prolonging the survival of men with established cardiovascular disease.

Many articles have supported the findings of the studies reported above. Berkman *et al.* (2000), writing one of the seminal works in this field, suggest mechanisms by which social networks may influence individual health status. Their explanations are drawn from a wide range of theory, from sociology to psychoanalysis. An important strand of Berkman *et al.*'s explanation is based on *attachment theory* (Bowlby 1969, 1973, 1980). Bowlby argues that the separation of infants from their mothers represented and unhealthy loss, resulting in a universal human need to form close affectionate bonds. According to attachment theory, the attached figure, generally the mother, creates a secure base from which the developing child can explore. Bowlby developed this proposal to the extent that he suggests that 'secure attachment provides an external ring of psychological protection which maintains the child's metabolism in a stable state similar to internal homeostatic mechanisms of blood pressure and temperature control'. It is these attachments formed in infancy that are said to provide a basis for attachment in adulthood. Individuals whose attachment in infancy is ambivalent or disorganised may be less able to form secure attachments in adulthood.

In the mid-twentieth century, anthropologists developed the concept of *social networks* to describe relationships that were independent of traditional, family, residential and social class groups. The analysis of social networks was concerned with understanding the patterns of ties between actors in a social system rather than on characteristics of the individuals themselves (Hall and Wellman, 1985). Thus, individual behaviour is largely determined by the social structure of the network rather than by the individual differences of its members. Berkman *et al.* (2000) identify a range of characteristics of social networks which are particularly influential:

- the range or number of network members
- the extent to which the members are connected to each other
- the degree to which they are defined on the basis of traditional structures, e.g. family, work or neighbourhood
- the extent to which individuals are similar within a network.

The characteristics of individual ties within the network include:

- frequency of contact
- the number of types of transactions of support provided by a set of ties
- the length of time an individual knows another
- the extent to which exchanges are reciprocated.

Berkman *et al.* (2000) postulate that social isolation disintegration and disconnectedness influence mortality by influencing the rate of ageing. They hypothesise that social isolation is 'a chronically stressful condition to which the organism responded by aging faster . . . the cumulative conditions which tend to occur in very old age [are] accelerated'.

There is biological support for this hypothesis. Rats that are handled frequently and early in life have been shown to recover faster from the effects of stressful stimuli than are rats which have never been handled, or which are experiencing maternal separation. Moreover, rats that were not handled showed age-related rises in hormones which were not found among rats that had experienced early handling.

It is very clear from the evidence available that direct pathways exist between people's social lives, personal interactions, sense of belonging and their biologically defined state of health or illness. This effect is extraordinarily powerful and should never be underestimated as an important determinant of a patient's general state of health.

Challenge 2: Applying changes in policy

Dorothy takes pleasure in bringing a small gift to the podiatrist each time she comes for an appointment. Recently, the employing authority issued a policy stating that 'Gifts from patients should not be accepted'. How do you deal with this without causing offence? The podiatrist will need to address this issue with tact and sensitivity. Whilst appreciative of the gifts that are brought, the podiatrist will need to abide by the new policy. Careful and diplomatic communication skills need to be employed.

Summary of important health psychology

The important psychological issues to be considered in the case of Dorothy are her positive traits and the positive effect of her strong family and social ties. Patients like Dorothy do not present a personal challenge in practice and fortunately are in the majority.

Implications for podiatric management

With effective home treatment, the fungal condition is entirely treatable. For detailed consideration of the treatment of dermatological conditions, refer to any dermatological textbook.

Chapter 20

Adolescence: the development and exploration of the self, self-esteem and social identity

Life is what happens while you are making other plans.

John Lennon

Adolescence is a time of physical and psychological change and includes the development and exploration of the self, self-esteem and social identity. It is a time when conventional approaches to medicine may be challenged and alternative approaches to treatment sought.

Sophie is a slightly overweight 17-year-old girl who was born with spina bifida. She is unable to walk unaided and spends much of her time in a wheelchair. She is a bright and lively girl who lives at home with her parents and her little brother, who is seven years old. Sophie aspires to a career in business administration, and when she left school at 16 she attended the local technical college, where she had enrolled on a secretarial course. Unfortunately, her health was not good during her first year at college, which resulted in her being often absent from her course. She had to intermit from the course but hopes to restart it at the beginning of the next academic year.

Her parents are unemployed and live on benefits, and they find looking after Sophie difficult and a full-time job. Her father has tried to find work, but is not committed to finding a job because he thinks he would only be slightly better off financially.

Sophie has peripheral neuropathy and has recently developed ulcers on her toes, where her shoes have been rubbing. She is eligible for podiatry treatment, but has a history of failing to attend for her appointments. Continuity of treatment is important for Sophie to treat her podiatric problems as and when they arise, and to monitor her condition. Maintenance of health is of utmost importance to enable her to be independent and achieve her goals and aspirations.

The podiatry clinic sends appointments, through the post, and leaves messages on Sophie's parents' answerphone. Sophie's father refuses to use the answer machine and will not listen to any messages that are left on it. He does not like opening 'official-looking envelopes' because he finds them intimidating. Sophie's mother runs an open house for all the local children, welcomes them in, befriends them all and enjoys dealing with their personal problems. Sophie's mother is slightly embarrassed about Sophie and finds it difficult having a handicapped daughter.

Sophie has recently been feeling disillusioned and 'let down' by allopathic (conventional) medicine and has developed an interest in complementary and homeopathic approaches. She is keen to know whether homeopathic preparations or complementary treatments would improve her health.

Factors influencing Sophie's behaviour

Spina bifida is a congenital deformity that usually begins between the fourth and sixth weeks of pregnancy. It is characterised by a defective closure in the vertebral column, of varying severity. There are two primary types of spina bifida: occulta and manifesta.

Spina bifida occulta is the milder form, in which the defective closure is beneath a layer of skin. It occurs when one or more of the vertebrae of the spine fail to fuse properly. There are generally no associated functional limitations.

Spina bifida manifesta has two common forms. In the rare but milder form, a skin-filled sac containing cerebral spinal fluid and nerve roots appears in the lower back. The most common and severe form is characterised by a failure of the spinal cord to form a tube and a portion of the undeveloped cord protrudes through the back. The cord forms a sac around it containing cerebrospinal fluid which may be covered by skin or simply by tissue and exposed nerves.

Ultimately, the severity of spina bifida is determined by the site of the protrusion and by which nerves are affected. Damage and symptoms occur when the spinal cord develops and the sac grows, damaging the surrounding nerves. Parts of the body corresponding to these damaged or undeveloped nerves will be impaired; there is a direct correlation between the area of the lesion and associated paralysis or other impairment.

Disabilities or functional limitations associated with spina bifida depend upon the location of the lesion and any associated nerve damage. The most common impairment is the partial or total paralysis of affected muscle groups. Since most lesions are found in the low thoracic, lumbar or sacral regions of the spine, the lower extremities, bowel and bladder function and sexual functions are most often involved. Ambulation must often be supplemented by wheelchairs and related aids. In more severe cases, the trunk and upper extremities are involved, further limiting independence in vocational and daily care skills.

In 1980, the World Health Organization attempted to standardise the classification of disability internationally, and suggested that *impairment* refers to physical or cognitive limitations that an individual may have, such as the inability to walk or speak. By contrast, *disability* relates to socially imposed restrictions, that is the system of social constraints that are imposed on those with impairments by the discriminatory practices of society. A *handicap* is a disadvantage resulting from impairment or a disability that limits or prevents the fulfilment of a role that is normal (depending on age, sex, and social and cultural factors) for that individual.

Disabled people, while not necessarily ill, may encounter a variety of social disadvantages as the result of stigma (Susman, 1994; Reynolds-Whyte and Ingstad, 1995), which makes a person different from others and thus be seen as less desirable (Breakey, 1997).

Body image is concerned with the way in which an individual perceives their own body and is predicated on an internal *model* of body shape and size (Fisher, 1973). This internal model is subjective rather than objective and may be altered by psychological states.

Western society has long been preoccupied with what it considers to be the perfect human form, although the exact nature of this form has changed across history. Whatever the contemporary fashion for body shape, deviation from it is generally viewed as undesirable (Breakey, 1997).

Despite her physical state, Sophie has great confidence in her own ability to succeed in her chosen career. The belief that one is able to achieve goals is often described as *self-efficacy*.

Self-efficacy was first described by Bandura in 1977, and is recognised as an important factor that may influence a wide range of health-related behaviours. To possess self-efficacy requires the belief in one's own competence; Sophie's self-efficacy in relation to her college work and career is strong, and it is very important that the podiatrist maximises the opportunity to draw on this strength.

The concept of self-efficacy has been examined in relation to disability and some of the psychological models described in Chapter 7. The World Health Organization (1980) distinguishes between the objective difficulties experienced by disabled people – impairment, the effects that impairment has on their ability to carry out everyday activities – and the effect of their impairment on fulfilling social roles – or handicap. This approach has led to an attempt to integrate impairment and disability in social cognition models. Hence, according to the so-called Integrated Model of Disability (Johnston, 1996), impairment directly influences the proximal components of the theory of planned behaviour, that is attitudes, subjective norms and perceived behavioural control. However, such suggestions have been forcefully rejected by disabled people themselves. The behaviours available to a disabled person are determined, at least in part, by the social environment and the degree to which society has made an investment in meeting their needs (Roberts *et al.*, 2001).

Roberts *et al.* suggest that the observation that various quality of life measures produce significantly different results when administered to the same group of disabled respondents (Ziebland *et al.*, 1993) confirms the inadequacy of defining *impairment* without considering the contribution of the social environment itself. Such observations reflect the broader distinction between medical models of disability, in which disability is defined by impairment of function, and social models of disability, in which disability is described in terms of the degree to which society can meet the needs of the disabled person.

In addition, Sophie is optimistic by nature and tends to latch on to any opportunity that she sees as having potential. This sometimes results in her accepting ideas uncritically and she may be regarded as slightly impressionable.

Sophie's parents provide such support as they are able. The way in which Sophie receives social support may be viewed in two ways: the support she feels she receives (*perceived social support*) and the support that she actually or potentially has (*structural social support*). In reality, perceived support is often more important than simply having structures in place for support to be given (Schaefer *et al.*, 1981).

Sophie does not feel particularly well supported by her parents. She considers herself to be more intelligent and better motivated than her father and resents the attention her mother gives to the other local children. Sophie is thus particularly vulnerable to the social influence of other people who are important in her life, notably her teachers, college friends and the range of health professionals involved in her care. Sophie's self-efficacy, independence and optimism combine to make her, on the one hand, keen to maximise her potential through hard work but, on the other hand, difficult to persuade to engage with her treatment unless she is thoroughly convinced of its efficacy.

Challenge 1: Complementary and alternative medicine

Sophie has recently visited a complementary medicine centre and feels that the treatment she received there was more beneficial than was her conventional treatment. Sophie is particularly interested in homeopathy and has consulted a practitioner regarding her ulcerated toes. There is limited evidence concerning the efficacy of homeopathic medicine in podiatry, although homeopathic remedies have been investigated as alternatives to some conventional podiatric treatments (Concha *et al.*, 1998; Khan, 2000a, 2000b).

However, Sophie is worried that you may be dismissive of all complementary therapies because she perceives you as being part of the 'medical establishment'.

Homeopathy, or homeopathic medicine, is a system of treatment that originated in the late eighteenth century. The name *homeopathy* is derived from two Greek words that mean 'like and disease'. Homeopathy is based on the idea that substances which produce symptoms of illness in healthy people will have a curative effect when given in very dilute quantities to sick people who exhibit those same symptoms.

Homeopathic remedies are believed to stimulate the body's own healing processes. Samuel Hahnemann (1755–1843), the founder of homeopathic medicine, used the Latin phrase *similia similibus curentur*, or 'let like be cured with like', to summarise the underlying principle of his system. By contrast, homeopaths use the term *allopathy*, or 'different than disease', to describe the use of drugs used in conventional medicine to oppose or counteract the symptom being treated.

The aim of homeopathy is the restoration of the body to homeostasis, or healthy balance, which is considered its natural state. The symptoms of a disease are regarded as the body's own defensive attempt to correct its imbalance, rather than as enemies to be defeated. Because a homeopath regards symptoms as positive evidence of the body's *inner intelligence*, he or she will prescribe a remedy designed to stimulate this internal curative process rather than suppress the symptoms.

Evidence-based practice dominates academic thinking and clinical medicine and has resulted in an increased emphasis on research findings and improved dissemination. However, since the end of the last century, there has been a small but discernible move among health care professionals to refer patients to, and to practise, complementary therapies for which there is little scientific evidence of their efficacy (Paterson and Britten, 1999).

Complementary medicine is clearly enjoying a popularity that would have seemed risible before the 1980s. Since then, there has clearly been a rapid growth in its popularity, both with conventional practitioners and among patients seeking treatment. An explanation of why these changes may have occurred is clearly of great interest to all professions based on notions of evidence-based care (Paterson and Britten, 1999).

A number of studies have attempted to address this issue by exploring the reasons patients give for seeking complementary treatments. In general practice, patients report the failure of conventional medicine to help their condition as their main motivation (Moore *et al.*, 1985; Vincent and Furnham, 1997). In addition, some patients report the use of complementary medicine as a supplement to orthodox medicine rather than as a replacement for it (Fulder and Munro, 1985; Thomas *et al.*, 1991).

Other work identifies five key factors which help to explain this change in thinking. These are: a positive evaluation of complementary treatment, the ineffectiveness of orthodox medicine, concerns about the adverse effects of orthodox medicine, poor communication skills among doctors and concerns about the availability of complementary medicine (Vincent and Furnham, 1997).

A criticism widely applied to many complementary therapies is that their effect is entirely due to suggestion. This effect is generally known as a *placebo*.

A placebo (Latin for *I shall please*) is any treatment which contains no known active ingredient yet which often has a measurable, observable or felt improvement in health that is reported by the patient.

The reason for why an inert substance should have a therapeutic effect is unknown. However, there is a very large body of literature which shows that placebos can be at least as effective as many active treatments.

Some researchers believe the placebo effect is entirely *psychological*, owing to a *belief* in the treatment resulting in a subjective *feeling* of improvement. Kirsch and Sapirstein, in a controversial paper, suggest that the effectiveness of Prozac and similar antidepressant drugs may be attributed almost entirely to a placebo effect. He analysed 19 clinical trials of antidepressants and concluded that the expectation of improvement, not adjustments in brain chemistry, accounted for 75% of the drugs' effectiveness (Kirsch and Sapirstein, 1998).

However, a person's beliefs and hopes about a treatment may have a significant biochemical effect. Both sensory experience and thoughts can affect neurochemistry. The body's neurochemical system affects and is affected by other biochemical systems, including the hormonal and immune systems. Thus, it is consistent with current knowledge that a person's hopeful attitude and beliefs may be very important to their physical well-being and recovery from injury or illness.

It is also possible that at least part of the placebo effect reflects an illness or injury taking its natural course of recovery. Because of the aggressive way in which many minor conditions are now treated, the natural history of many ailments is unclear. It is thus possible that a condition which appears to respond to a placebo may have resolved itself without treatment in any case. Moreover, many disorders, pains and illnesses wax and wane. What is observed as a placebo effect may, in many cases, represent a natural regression to the mean.

However, none of these proposals is adequate to fully explain the magnitude and iniquitousness of the placebo effect, and this remains a particularly interesting area for active research.

Perhaps most importantly, much of what has been labelled a placebo effect may occur as a result of the way in which therapy is given, that is the process of administering therapy (Roberts *et al.*, 1993). Many consider the touching, the caring, the attention and other interpersonal communication along with the hopefulness and encouragement provided by the therapist to be key factors which alter the mood of the patient. This in turn triggers physical changes, such as the release of endorphins, which reduces stress. This reduction in stress prevents or slows down further harmful physical changes from occurring.

The *process of treatment* hypothesis may explain how the therapies offered by many complementary practitioners are often effective. It may also explain the efficacy of treatments initially thought to work by a given mechanism that is subsequently disproved.

Whether Sophie continues with her homeopathy is not an issue for the podiatrist. More important is that she continues to be monitored and provided with evidence-based podiatric treatment.

Challenge 2: How would you convince Sophie of the necessity to attend her podiatry appointments?

The most important factor in achieving this aim lies in the relationship that the podiatrist develops with Sophie. The podiatrist must respect Sophie's views about her chosen therapy. Respect is not the mere tolerance of a different viewpoint; respect requires recognition of equality between the values of the patient and the professional. It is this equality which is critical in maintaining Sophie's willingness to continue both in the relationship with the podiatrist and with treatment.

Summary of important health psychology

Adolescence is a time of significant physical and psychological change and development and the exploration of the self. It is a crucial stage in the development of self-esteem and social identity. An understanding of these processes and the importance of social support in adolescence will enable the podiatrist to build an effective therapeutic relationship with Sophie. In order to do this, the podiatrist must recognise that although Sophie's views may differ from his/her own they are no less valid and should be treated with appropriate respect.

Implications for podiatric management

The first priority for podiatric management is to treat the infection and heal any ulceration. In parallel with this baseline, measures should be taken of neurological and vascular status, and of skin integrity, against which ongoing monitoring can be undertaken. Prevention of recurrent ulceration centres on the removal of pressure. Sensitivity must be used when recommending footwear, acknowledging that Sophie is likely to want to wear fashionable shoes.

Chapter 21

Behavioural change

It is not I who become addicted; it is my body.
Jean Cocteau

Podiatrists may be involved in reinforcing the benefits of changing behaviour. In this character, the podiatrist is faced with advising George Archer of the benefits of giving up smoking. The character of George explains why it is so difficult to give up smoking and provides a model to explain the process.

George is a 60-year-old builder who is currently working in his own business, but is looking forward to retiring shortly. He has worked continuously since his apprenticeship began when he was 15 years old, and he is very proud of his achievements. His business is well respected throughout the local community and he is perceived by his friends and colleagues as a very honest and straightforward individual. He has two grown-up sons and three small grandchildren, of whom he is very proud.

George has been an insulin-dependent diabetic for 45 years and is well controlled. He eats a sensible diet, and drinks alcohol in moderation. George has smoked cigarettes since he was a teenager. He used to smoke heavily but has recently cut down to around 15 cigarettes a day. He suffers from early peripheral vascular disease and has a mild degree of lower-limb neuropathy. He has been attending the podiatry clinic for six months for routine care and monitoring. Continued use of tobacco is strongly associated with the development of peripheral vascular disease, which may result in ulceration and gangrene.

In order to prevent development of the negative consequences of his condition, it is essential that George stop smoking.

Factors influencing George's behaviour

George is a man who believes that hard work results in a good quality of life. His status and position are important to him, and he enjoys the respect that he receives from his friends and colleagues.

The blood supply to George's feet, particularly to his toes, is compromised by his diabetes. Nicotine is a potent vasoconstrictor, which exacerbates his problem. If the blood supply to George's feet continues to be reduced in this way, it is likely that his healing ability will be impaired and ultimately his toes may become gangrenous. In addition, smoking is also associated with large blood vessel disease and coronary heart disease.

Coronary artery disease is the most common form of heart disease. It results from the gradual build-up of hardened deposits called *plaques* in the arteries supplying the heart muscle and is called *atherosclerosis*. Over time, the plaques, which consist of deposits of fat, cholesterol, calcium and other cellular particulate from the blood, constrict the coronary arteries, resulting in a diminished blood flow to the heart. This reduced blood flow to the heart can result in chest pain (*angina*) and complete blockage of an artery can lead to ischaemia of the myocardium (a heart attack).

Many people are unaware that they are developing coronary artery disease. The disease often develops slowly and in the absence of symptoms, over a period of decades. It is not uncommon for a heart attack to be the first sign that an individual has the disease.

Diseases of the heart and circulatory system (*cardiovascular disease*, or CVD) are the main cause of death in the United Kingdom, accounting for over 250 000 deaths in 1998 (British Heart Foundation Statistics, 2000). This accounts for one in three deaths in the United Kingdom.

The main forms of CVD are coronary heart disease (CHD) and stroke. About half of all deaths from CVD are from CHD and about a quarter are from stroke. CHD by itself is the most common cause of death in the United Kingdom. One in four men and one in five women die from the disease. CHD caused over 135 000 deaths in the United Kingdom in 1998.

The rate of premature death from CHD in the United Kingdom is 58% higher for male manual workers than it is for male non-manual workers. The premature death rate from CHD for female manual workers is more than twice that for female non-manual workers.

Overall, the rate of death from CHD is falling across all social groups for both men and women in the United Kingdom. However, the death rate among men is falling faster in non-manual workers than it is in manual workers. The result is that the class-related difference in death rates is widening. It is estimated that each year 5000 lives and 47 000 working years are lost in men aged 20–64 years owing to social class inequalities in CHD death rates. Just under one in three of all deaths under 65 years resulting from social class inequalities are due to CHD.

Diabetes substantially increases an individual's risk of developing CHD. Men with non-insulin-dependent (type 2) diabetes have a two- to fourfold greater annual risk of CHD, with an even higher (three- to fivefold) risk in women with type 2 diabetes (Garcia et al., 1974).

Around 3% of adult men and women in England have diabetes (Stamler et al., 1993). The prevalence of diabetes increases with age: those aged 65–74 are around 10 times more likely as those aged 25–34 to have the disease. Overall, diabetes is more prevalent in men than in women (3.3% versus 2.5%), although women aged 16–24 are more likely to have diabetes than men of a similar age.

As in many countries, diabetes is increasing in the United Kingdom. Since 1991, prevalence has increased by around two-thirds among men and by a quarter among women. About two-thirds of people with diabetes die of some form of heart or blood vessel disease.

In type 1 diabetes, the beta cells of the pancreas produce little or no insulin. Insulin is a hormone that allows the sugar glucose to enter body cells. Once glucose enters a cell, it is used as fuel. Without adequate insulin, glucose builds up in the bloodstream instead of going into the cells. The body is unable to use glucose for energy, despite high levels of it in the bloodstream. This causes symptoms such as excessive thirst, increased urine output and feelings of hunger. Within five to 10 years of diagnosis, the insulin-producing cells of the pancreas are destroyed, and no more insulin is produced.

Type 1 diabetes can occur at any age, but usually occurs before 30 years of age. Symptoms are usually more severe and occur rapidly with this type of diabetes. People with this condition require insulin to live.

The exact cause of type 1 diabetes is not known; however, a family history of diabetes, viruses that injure the pancreas and destruction of insulin-making cells by the body's immune system may play causative roles. Risk factors for type 1 diabetes include immune system diseases, viral infections and a family history of diabetes.

Insulin-dependent diabetes accounts for 3% of all new cases of diabetes each year. There is one new case per 7000 children each year. The number of new cases decreases after age 20.

People who smoke have a risk of heart attack that is more than twice that of non-smokers. Cigarette smoking is the biggest risk factor for sudden cardiac death. Smokers who have a heart attack are more likely to die as a result and to do so suddenly (within an hour of onset). People who smoke cigars or pipes have an increased risk of death from coronary heart disease (and possibly stroke) compared to non-smokers, but cigarette smokers carry the highest risk. Constant exposure to other people's smoke increases the risk of heart disease even for non-smokers.

It is estimated that about 20% of deaths from CHD in men and 17% of deaths from CHD in women are due to smoking, but that only 0.5% of deaths from CHD in the United Kingdom could be avoided if the Government's new targets for smoking prevalence (26% by 2005 and 24% by 2010) were to be met (British Heart Foundation Statistics, 2000).

Gangrene is the term for the death of tissue (*necrosis*). There are several potential causes, including interruption of the blood supply, infection with certain bacteria and damage from freezing. Gangrene in an extremity is due to an interruption of the blood supply to that limb. If the involved tissue remains free of infection, it shrivels up and becomes dry and dark in colour (*dry gangrene*). If the dead tissue becomes infected, it becomes moist (*wet gangrene*). Antibiotics may be used to treat the infection.

Important psychological theory

Why is smoking so difficult to give up? Many thousands of studies have been written on the psychology of cigarette smoking. Nicotine is an addictive substance, but psychological dependence may often be more important than chemical addiction. The process by which many people stop smoking has been the subject of much discussion.

One of the most influential theories that have been used to understand smoking behaviour is the Transtheoretical, or Stages of Change, Model proposed by Prochaska and DiClemente (1983). The model suggests a circular structure, as shown in Figure 21.1 below.

A person in the pre-contemplation phase may be described as the *contented smoker*. At some point, most smokers begin to consider giving

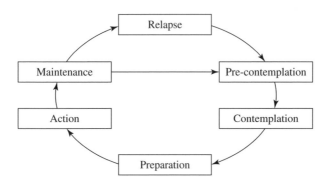

Figure 21.1 The Transtheoretical Model. (Adapted from Prochaska and DiClemente, 1983.)

up smoking and by so doing move into the *contemplation phase*. It is at this point that thoughts about the benefits of not smoking are first seen to be attractive. From this phase, the would-be ex-smoker moves into a *preparation stage*; this stage is characterised by activities such as disposing of ashtrays, lighters, making a date to stop etc. If this is successful, the individual shifts to the *action stage* and quits smoking altogether. From this stage, the individual may remain abstinent or may relapse, from which the whole cycle may begin at a later date, or he/she may remain as a smoker in the pre-contemplation stage.

Limitations of the Transtheoretical Model

Several authors have described limitations to this model (for example Lucas and Lloyd, 2005). First, it has been suggested that there is little empirical evidence for the existence of the distinct stages the model proposes, let alone that they exist in the circular order suggested by Prochaska and DiClemente.

An illustration of this criticism may be seen in relation to smoking behaviour. In this domain, the model's stages are often defined as follows:

- **Pre-contemplation**: one who is not contemplating quitting in the next six months.
- **Preparation**: one who is planning to quit in next 30 days and who has made at least one attempt lasting one day or more in the last 12 months.
- **Contemplation**: everybody else.

Even these basic algorithms present problems. First, the classification is arbitrary: why not three months and seven days instead of six months and 30 days? Second, the stage construct is, in Fishbein and Ajzen's terminology, a composite of intention and behaviour. More seriously, Sutton (1996) points out that, according to the model, a smoker cannot be in the preparation stage unless they have made a recent quit attempt. It follows that the first time they tried to quit they must have done so without being in the preparation stage. A smoker can thus never be 'prepared' for his/her first quit attempt. Similarly, Stockwell, (1996) asks:

> how reliably different are smokers who are 'contemplating quitting smoking in the next six months' versus those who are not? What does it mean to be contemplating such a thing? Does one have to be contemplating this now, five minutes ago, some time today or in the past week? Surely every smoker these days contemplates quitting at regular intervals?

A more detailed criticism of the Stages of Change Model in predicting smoking cessation is provided by Farkas *et al.* (1996). They found that when stage of change was used as a stand-alone predictor, smokers in 'preparation' at baseline were more likely than those in 'pre-contemplation' to be abstinent at follow-up. However, when stage membership was combined with measures of pharmacological addiction, the former no longer predicted cessation. Moreover, occasional versus daily smoking, number of cigarettes smoked and lifetime number of quits discriminated abstinence much better at follow-up than did stages of change; the overall prediction by the Stages of Change Model yielded 55%, whilst overall prediction by the addition model yielded nearly 70%. Farkas and his colleagues conclude that:

> our results question the validity of the stages of change construct as a predictor of smoking cessation. Although smokers in the preparation stage at baseline showed higher rates of cessation one to two years later, we observed no difference in follow-up cessation rates between those in the contemplation stage and those in the pre-contemplation stage at baseline. Furthermore, stage of change was not an independent predictor when used in the multivariate analysis with other predictors.

Other researchers are even more explicit in their criticism. For example, Pierce *et al.* (1996) found no significant difference in quitting history by stage of change in a longitudinal study of over 2000 smokers. They conclude:

> While we agree that the stage of change model has had considerable historical importance in getting clinicians to accept behaviour change as a process, this does not mean that it has successfully ousted earlier paradigms in health promotion. Before we put any theory on such a pedestal we should carefully scrutinise its performance compared with the previously accepted theories. This is particularly so for a model that has been accused of achieving prominence with a relative absence of scientific support for its validity.

It is certainly true that this model has, as Pierce *et al.* suggest, been 'put on a pedestal'. By October 1997, a UK training programme called Helping People Change had over 500 trainers throughout England. These trainers taught a course with a 12-hour core, plus several additional four-hour modules, based on Prochaska and DiClemente's Stages of Change Model. The main target audience for this training were Primary Care professionals and allied workers. Well over four and a half thousand practitioners were trained by 1997.

It is well established that many negative health behaviours, notably smoking, a sedentary lifestyle and a high-fat diet are more common among people in lower socio-economic groups. It is therefore unsurprising to note that the prevalence of many diseases including coronary heart disease and some cancers follows a similar pattern (Table 21.1).

Table 21.1 The relative risk of death from coronary heart disease according to employment grade.

Relative risk (log scale)	Administrative classes	Professional/ Executive classes	Clerical	Other
Cholesterol, smoking, other	1.0	0.3	0.9	1.4
Unexplained	0	1.8	2.3	2.6
Total	**1.0**	**2.1**	**3.2**	**4.0**

Source: Adapted from Wilkinson, 1997.

However, it is important to understand that the socio-economic gradient reported in both morbidity and mortality cannot be adequately explained solely in terms of differences in health-related behaviours. The work of Marmot *et al.* (1991) involving a sample of British civil servants clearly demonstrates that traditional targets of health promotion campaigns (for example smoking, exercise and diet) only contribute a minor amount of variance in the observed relationship of morbidity and mortality to social class. When such variables are controlled, the great majority of social class variation in coronary heart disease and other causes of mortality remains.

Other investigators have suggested that this variation may be due to a wide range of social factors, such as stress, poorer social support and increased risk of social isolation, which operate on psychological, neurological and immunological levels.

In George's case, it is clearly important that he stop smoking. He is fortunate that he has a strong and supportive family network and a stable marriage. These are resources which will be an invaluable asset in his attempts to give up tobacco.

Challenge 1: How could you capitalise on George's stable social environment to facilitate his attempts to stop smoking?

In order for the podiatrist to influence George's behaviour, it is important for the podiatrist to identify at which stage in the cycle George is currently situated. The aim is then to help George to move on to the next stage of the cycle. For example, it would be inappropriate to discuss issues such as nicotine replacement therapy (NRT) with George if he is still in pre-contemplation. In this case, it would be more helpful to encourage George to consider the benefits of stopping smoking, both in terms of his own health and the potential effect on his family. At this stage, it might be helpful if George were exposed to a cost-benefit analysis of his smoking behaviour, which may be facilitated by the podiatrist. If George is in the contemplation stage, it will be more helpful to discuss practical issues such as setting a quit date, strategies to replace smoking and NRT.

The preparation stage includes such issues as determining a date for quitting, the best circumstances for George to quit and enrolling family and friends into helping him stop. The action stage begins when George stops smoking completely. If this stage is sustained, he moves into the *maintenance period*. During all of these stages, it is important that George be encouraged and positive reinforcement be provided. It is often useful to encourage people to substitute cigarette smoking with a more healthy activity.

Should George relapse at any stage, it is important that the podiatrist try to help to move him on to the contemplation stage again. For many smokers, the first attempts to give up can be unsuccessful, and reinforcement and encouragement are vital to enable eventual success, but it should be noted that repeated encouragement should not be seen by George as nagging.

The podiatrist's ability to judge accurately the current stage at which George is located is clearly dependent upon building a successful therapeutic relationship. Therapeutic relationships are discussed in detail in Chapter 5.

Challenge 2: What other assistance can be offered to George in order to help him stop smoking?

There are many reasons why giving up smoking is difficult but one cause is relatively straightforward to address. Among the many constituents of tobacco smoke, it is nicotine that is the most powerfully habit forming. It is well established that most people who quit smoking successfully do so by stopping completely and suddenly as opposed to attempting to cut down before abstinence. Reducing the number of cigarettes that the individual smokes in a day is invariably accompanied by the individual inhaling more often and more deeply so that his/her blood nicotine level is maintained. Smokers have been shown to be able to titrate their blood nicotine levels very accurately by this means. It is therefore very helpful if the withdrawal symptoms induced by abstinence can be alleviated. Such relief is effectively offered by any of the variety of nicotine replacement products now available over the counter. It is important that these products be used in the directed way. Nicotine is excreted from the body quite rapidly and it is important that patients do not use such preparations for excessive periods or take more than the dose recommended. It is therefore important for all health professionals to have an understanding of the NRT products when offering support to smokers wishing to quit.

While the combined effect of support from a health professional and NRT can significantly improve people's chances of successfully giving up smoking, it is important for the podiatrist to be aware that even with the most effective interventions run by the most skilled professionals there are still very high relapse rates. Podiatrists should not feel that their efforts have failed if George starts smoking again. Most smokers who quit have a history of a number of relapses before they become permanently abstinent.

Summary of important health psychology

Giving up smoking is a complex and difficult process for many people. A number of models have been employed to attempt to explain how this process operates. The Transtheoretical, or Stages of Change, Model (Prochaska and DiClemente, 1983) provides a useful framework within which the podiatrist may approach George's smoking and provide support to help him quit.

Implications for podiatric management

The aims for George are that his condition is carefully monitored and that any initial signs of deterioration are noted. Therefore, arrangements should be made for review of all assessments. Routine nail and skin care may be undertaken by a podiatry assistant under delegated supervision of the podiatrist responsible for George's management. Of great importance are foot health education and the provision of information regarding prevention of any podiatric complications associated with peripheral vascular and neuropathic conditions.

Chapter 22

The influence of religion and spirituality on health

He's not the kind you have to wind up on Sundays.

Ian Anderson

Neil Anderson is a 38-year-old social worker. He has spent many years involved in working with young people both in this country and overseas. He is unmarried, largely as a result of devoting all of his spare time to voluntary organisations. Neil is a profoundly religious man and his beliefs drive him to devote his life to benefiting other people. He has recently returned from at trip to Africa, where he has spent the last year engaged in development projects that have provided clean water, sanitation and basic education to a village of underprivileged children and adults.

He presented at the clinic complaining of sore, discoloured and weeping areas of skin between his toes and with pustules on the arch of the foot. This presentation is indicative of a fungal infection probably with overlying bacterial involvement. Neil is a very charming and likeable man who is very willing to be involved in his treatment in principle, but fears that he may be unable to attend to his treatment as diligently as required. He is an unassuming individual who gives the impression of having limited self-confidence; he gives the impression that it would be alien to his nature to act assertively. Neil's lack of assertiveness is a function of his religious beliefs and a conviction that his actions and future are solely a result of and subservient to God's will.

Currently, these beliefs have led him to plan a further trip to Africa, where standards of hygiene are poor and access to pharmaceutical services is extremely limited. Nevertheless, Neil is adamant that, because he is doing what God has planned for him, his faith will ensure his well-being. Not unreasonably, Neil points out to the podiatrist that the needs of the people he is helping are much greater than his own needs and that his podiatric condition is trivial in comparison to the conditions in which they live.

Factors influencing Neil's behaviour

Psychologists regard the domain of spirituality with a powerful ambivalence which is as old as the discipline's roots. Freud considered any religious inclination to be diagnostic of immaturity. Pressured by his Jewish background, he married the granddaughter of the Chief Rabbi of Hamburg in a Jewish ceremony, but was so opposed to its tenets that he considered converting to Protestantism in order to avoid it. Palmer (1997) notes that Freud's vitriolic atheism was based on intellectual, formal principles. While Freud maintained his cultural identity in what he described a 'life-affirming Judaism', he rejected both religious belief and ritual practices. In a letter to Jung on 2nd January 1910, he argued that:

> It has occurred to me that the ultimate basis of man's need for religion is *infantile helplessness*, which is so much greater in man than in animals. After infancy he cannot conceive of a world without parents, and makes for himself a just God and a kindly nature, the two worst anthropomorphic falsifications he could have imagined . . .

Conversely, Jung (particularly later in life) became increasingly convinced that *denial* of a spiritual nature in humanity was indicative of *incomplete individuation*. Jung (1928, 1943) uses this term to mean a process in which a person:

> [becomes] an 'in-dividual', and, in so far as 'individuality' embraces our inner-most, last, and incomparable unique-ness, it also implies becoming one's own self. We could therefore translate individuation as 'coming to self-hood' or 'self-realization.

From Neil's perspective, carrying out God's will is the guiding principle in his life and one which overrides any considerations of personal well-being. At both a religious and a psychological level, this belief is an essential component of Neil's *raison d'être*.

Among academics, the struggle for the emergence of psychology as an independent discipline has further polarised opinion regarding spirituality and human well-being. In an effort to free itself from what some viewed as the unscientific background of psychoanalysis, psychology has striven tirelessly to establish itself as a science. This effort has manifested itself in many ways. Psychology graduates often tend to be more numerate than those from other disciplines in the social sciences; quantitative studies constitute the great majority of the subject's literature; statistical software designed specifically for psychologists is as at least as sophisticated as any developed for engineering or the natural sciences.

Levin (1994) suggests that other factors are also involved. First, while many studies in psychology and epidemiology have reported a link between religiosity and health outcomes, very few of them actually set out to explore this relationship intentionally. Generally, the occasional measure of religiosity has been 'added to the mix' of variables examined in relation to outcomes such as cardiovascular disease and various cancers. Levin notes that

> Findings bearing on religion–health linkages were then buried in tables, often without comment in either text or abstract, and usually without reference to similar findings from other studies.

Second, Levin suggests that ideological and institutional barriers in medicine have discouraged the dissemination of positive findings. Levin and Vanderpool (1989) summarise the situation thus:

> Western biomedicine, of which epidemiology is a part, is still wrestling with a mind–body dualism that defies consensus; thus for most epidemiologists, any resolution of a mind–body–spirit pluralism is simply beyond consideration.

Despite attitudes ranging from indifference through ambivalence to hostility in the medical establishment, several hundred studies concerning the link between religiosity and health do exist. In the late nineteenth century, John Shaw Billings noted that religious affiliation appeared to operate as a protective factor in differential rates of morbidity and mortality among different social groups (Billings, 1891). A hundred years before Sir Douglas Black embarrassed the government of the day by identifying health inequalities in the United Kingdom, the French sociologist Emile Durkheim identified systematic differences in suicide rates between Jews, Catholics and Protestants (Durkheim, 1897). Since then, several reviews of epidemiological studies have been produced which have yielded similar results. One of the earliest of these, by Jenkins (1971), is notable because of its publication in the *New England Journal of Medicine*, which prepared the way for many others in mainstream medical journals. Yet perhaps the most influential work appeared 17 years later in the *Southern Medical Journal* (Byrd, 1988), in which the author reported the apparently positive results of prayer on coronary care outcomes. The study resulted in so much controversy that it provoked a flurry of editorials and essays in journals ranging from the *Journal of Family Practice* to *Social Science and Medicine*.

Levin (1994) traces the more recent literature in this field and notes that studies of religion and health have appeared in most leading medical journals including *Journal of the American Medical Association*, the

Lancet, the *American Journal of Public Health* and the *American Journal of Epidemiology*.

Given the long and respected list of publications which have reported at least associations between spirituality and health, the question arises as to why the widespread dissemination of such data has not resulted in any meaningful response from health promotion workers. We would suggest that the answer might involve a failure to distinguish between organised, formal religion and human spirituality in general. The understandable reticence of statutory funding bodies to become involved with religion and its associated social and political complications has, in our view, resulted in an extensive and important area of human experience remaining in receipt of very little attention from health promotion theorists and virtually none from practitioners.

Yet such reticence is hardly evidence-based. In an early review of such studies, Levin and Schiller (1987) concluded that

> generally speaking, religiosity, however operationalised, seems to exert a salutary effect on health, regardless of the outcomes or diseases or types of rates which are examined.

In addition, Levin and Schiller (1987) report two other major findings. When comparing religious groups, there appears to be a relatively lower risk of illness among adherents to more behaviourally strict religions or denominations. For example, Mormons, Seventh-Day Adventists, Orthodox Jews and clergy of all faiths appear to be at lower risk of morbidity and mortality than do more behaviourally 'liberal' people. Second, within religious denominations, there is a trend towards better health, lower morbidity and lower mortality rates among people with higher levels of religiosity. Rates of religious attendance are inversely linked to a strikingly wide range of illnesses, including hypertension, trichomoniasis, cervical cancer, tuberculosis, neonatal mortality and many other conditions, as well as to overall mortality rates. Levin and Schiller note that this relationship is found in all faiths: their review includes all major religious groups, as well as Sephardic Jews, Benedictine monks, Baptist clergy, Adventists, Mormons and Zen Buddhists. Moreover, this relationship persisted, however the notion of *level of religiosity* was operationalised.

Clearly, such findings need to be assessed critically. Levin and Schiller (1987) argue that it is necessary to consider a number of distinct issues before any real relationship between religiosity and health may be viewed to be likely. First, can such an apparent relationship be due solely to chance effects or to biased studies? Levin and Schiller suggest that such causes alone are unlikely for several reasons. First, hundreds of published studies overwhelmingly report statistically significant positive associations between religiosity and health. Most of these are epidemiological studies of entire populations or of randomised samples. Second, there has been considerable diversity in the design of the studies involved, including prospective, retrospective, cohort and case-control studies, in studies both of children and of adults. Moreover, many of these studies have been multi-ethnic in nature, including samples of US white and black Protestants, European Catholics, Indian Parsees, Zulus from South Africa, Japanese Buddhists and Israeli Jews. Third, Levin and Schiller's review identifies consistent results from studies drawn from a 50-year period between the 1930s and the 1980s. Finally, such studies have been applied to a wide range of physical conditions, including both self-limiting acute illnesses and fatal, chronic diseases. Consistent associations have been noted in relation to illnesses with long, short or absent latency periods between exposure, diagnosis and mortality. It thus seems improbable that any observed relationship between religiosity and health can be explained solely in terms of chance or bias effects.

The second issue to be considered, according to Levin and Schiller, before accepting that there is a relationship between religiosity and health is whether it is possible (and perhaps likely) that people who hold strong religious beliefs may behave differently to others, particularly in terms of the health-related behaviours that are the traditional targets of health promotion activity: smoking, excessive alcohol use, drug misuse, an over-rich diet, lack of exercise and liberal sexual behaviour. Yet the congruence of many religious and health-related behaviours may suggest that compartmentalisation into 'religious' and 'health-related' behaviours is artificial. This is clearly the case in relation to Neil. Neil neither drinks nor smokes and his diet is modest. However, his beliefs lead him to consider his own physical health to be not only secondary to the needs of other people but also entirely a matter of God's will. He is apt to view caring for himself as self-indulgent and inappropriate.

Third, heredity may be an influence. Some religious communities rarely marry outside their own faith, a practice which may serve to maintain a 'healthy gene pool', thus reducing the prevalence of certain diseases in those groups. There is some evidence to support this suggestion. For example, a high incidence of Tay-Sachs Disease has been reported among Ashkenazic Jews, as has a similarly high incidence of hypercholesterolaemia among Dutch Reformed Afrikaners and of sickle cell anaemia among (predominantly black) US National Baptist Convention members. By contrast, there is a correspondingly low incidence of sickle cell anaemia among (predominantly white) US Southern Baptist Convention members. Clearly, these differences are likely to be due to the genetic characteristics of different religious groups, rather than theological differences; however, such characteristics do not account for the effects of changes in religious affiliation, or for the marked overall effect of religiosity versus non-religiosity.

Fourth, it is conceivable that frequent religious involvement has salutogenic 'side effects' which are psychosocial in origin. Many possible mechanisms have been considered (independent of considerations of religiosity), and some of these are discussed elsewhere in this book. Perhaps the most extensively investigated is social support, both in material and practical terms. However, other studies have suggested beneficial effects of possessing a sense of belonging and of order. Antonovsky (1979) developed the notion of *Sense of Coherence* (SOC), which he suggests has three component factors, namely comprehensibility (the extent to which an individual sees his/her life as meaningful and comprehensible), manageability (the extent to which problems are seen as manageable) and meaningfulness (the degree to which life is seen as having some king of meaning). Neil's religious beliefs are a vital source of his SOC and any treatment that is planned for him must take this into consideration. Irrespective of the podiatrist's views on religion or spirituality, Neil's beliefs are central to his behaviour, and this must be treated with respect and understanding.

Clearly, religious belief and ritual may serve to engender a sense of coherence among practitioners, which is entirely congruent with Antonovsky's components of SOC. On the other hand, it is possible that religiosity may have an opposite effect. The dogma associated with some religious traditions manifestly encourages guilt, low self-esteem and doubt, in addition to a social ordering which many people would find oppressive.

Nevertheless, a number of studies have explored Antonovsky's concept of SOC, and have noted a relationship between a high SOC and a low level of illness. For example, Bäckman (1990, 1991) reports results from two Finnish studies where items from Antonovsky's scale were related to good health, although the direction of this relationship is unclear as both of these were cross-sectional studies. Nevertheless, longitudinal studies have also reported a relationship between SOC and both physical and mental health (Dahlin *et al.*, 1990; Kalimo and Vuori, 1990, 1991).

It is important to note that most of these studies have approached SOC from a psychological frame of reference. Antonovsky, by contrast, views SOC as a social concept; thus SOC grows among people brought up in a socio-economically stable environment with *clearly defined norms and values* (such as among religious groups). Clearly, given Antonovsky's definition, a reasonable beginning for any analysis of the distribution of SOC would be those commonly agreed demographic variables known to influence health status: sex, age and social class.

Lundberg and Nyström Peck (1994) explored the relationship of SOC to demographic variables and to ill health in the Swedish population. In a sample of 3872 people aged 25–75, they found that the risk of circulatory problems was 80% higher in respondents with low SOC, while such people were at a 300% increased risk of psychological problems. When all other known risk factors were controlled, individuals with low reported SOC remained at a 50% increased risk of circulatory disease and a 250% increased risk of psychological distress. Lundberg and Nyström Peck conclude that the observed relationship is likely to be causal, that having a high SOC may be protective against circulatory and psychological problems and, importantly, that that SOC is both internally and externally determined.

Fifth, Levin and Schiller consider the psychodynamics of belief systems, religious rites and faith, particularly in relation to placebo effects. The combination of a sense of purpose, the easing of fear and uncertainty and a strong belief in the salutary effects of religion may all combine to produce health-enhancing results.

Yet the link between religiosity and health may still not be causal. Hill (1965) proposes a list of nine qualities in a relationship, the presence of which at least may be considered supportive of causality. Levin (1994) employs this framework to consider the relationship between religiosity and health outcomes, and found seven of the criteria (strength, consistency, temporality, a biological gradient, plausibility, coherence and analogy) to be met. While one of the remaining criteria, experimental evidence, is provided by Byrd's (1988) study of prayer on coronary care outcomes, the study remains controversial, and differs from other studies in that it involves people other than the subjects themselves. The final criterion, specificity, requires the independent variable to have an effect on a specific dependent variable (in this case, on specific disease). As religiosity appears to have an effect on a wide range of health-related outcomes, his criterion is not met by definition, rather than by weakness of the association.

Of course, it is entirely possible that a combination of many factors may explain some of the apparently salutogenic effects of religiosity via psycho-neuroimmunologic pathways. However, if this were true, Levin's (1994) argument elegantly articulates the pointlessness (in our view) of *explanation* without translating such findings into intervention:

> For example, while there is greater mortality among lonely widows and single men, it is hardly sufficient to say that this is fully explained by psycho-neuroimmunologic factors, even though the process of mortality is reducible to certain physiological and biochemical events. Granting explanatory primacy to one particular level of the human system (cultural, social, psychological, organ systems, cellular, molecular, etc.) is arbitrary; human biology is itself 'explained' by the activity of molecules and ultimately, to paraphrase Democritus, everything is just atoms and empty space. Yet no-one would suggest that research in atomic physics will yield the best approach for improving the life expectancy of lonely or bereaved people.

Whether the nature of an undeniable relationship between religiosity and health becomes clarified by future research is, in our pragmatic view, irrelevant. Historically, some form of spirituality may be seen as a basic human characteristic, which manifests itself in culturally moderated forms. Moreover, its effects on health outcomes appear to be very pronounced. For example, Comstock and Partridge's (1972) study shows the relative risk of infrequent church attendance to have a relative risk ratio of 3.9 for certain diseases. By contrast, King and Locke (1980) report standardised mortality ratios among the clergy as low as 9 for some causes of death. If only a fraction of these results was attributable solely to spirituality, they would remain effects comparable in magnitude with the more familiar targets of health promotion activity.

Challenge 1: Given the apparent health benefits of religious belief, how can the podiatrist persuade Neil to consider his own welfare as important?

In order for Neil to fully appreciate the requirement to treat and resolve the acute fungal and bacterial infection and then to prevent a reoccurrence of the condition, it is necessary to understand his personal perspective. To Neil, personal welfare is a matter entirely secondary to the welfare of other people, whom he sees as being more needy and worthy of care. Clearly, the people who he seeks to help have much more serious and ongoing needs than Neil has himself, and this must be acknowledged by the podiatrist. Nevertheless, Neil needs to be fit enough in order to be effective in his work in Africa and this is dependent upon the successful treatment of his condition. Engaging Neil in his treatment regime is dependent upon both *demonstrating* an understanding of his perspective and *emphasising* the podiatrist's desire to enable Neil to be in the best position to help the people he will encounter.

Challenge 2: What professional dilemma does this present to the podiatrist?

The case of Neil Anderson provides a good example of the distinction to made between compliance and concordance, discussed in Chapter 5. It is entirely possible that following his return to Africa, Neil's circumstances will lead him to either cease treatment altogether or, at best, modify his treatment as he will become completely absorbed in his work. Moreover, any medication which Neil takes with him or that he is able to access whilst in Africa may find its way to helping others rather than Neil himself. While it will be helpful for the podiatrist to provide as much therapeutic help to Neil whilst he remains in contact, there is a need to *agree to differ* and be realistic about the likelihood of treatment outcomes. Different people have different priorities, which may not always accord with professional objectives, and these values must be respected.

Summary of important health psychology

When considering the important health psychology theories that may be associated with Neil's situation, it may be useful to consider the health locus of control theory previously mentioned in Chapter 8 and Chapter 19. The theory would suggest that Neil does not believe that his life is under his own control but that circumstances arise because of a divinity. The theory of SOC is also important in this case, because of the health benefits which belong to a community of like-minded others.

Implications for podiatric management

It is important in the management of Neil to establish a timeline which can be agreed with him. The acute phase must be aggressively treated with systemic antibiotics, topical antiseptics and antifungal agents whilst awaiting results of laboratory investigations as to causative organisms. It may be beneficial to suggest potassium permanganate footbaths, which have additional antiseptic, antiperspirant and deodorant properties. In the longer term, specific antimicrobials need to be prescribed until such time that the symptoms have been eradicated for at least three weeks. This is often a challenge, as many patients believe themselves to be cured, but fungal spores may be dormant and when conditions become optimum for their development the infection may become active once more. Of great importance is prevention of re-infection, especially since Neil proposes to travel abroad once more. Footwear, including socks (there are now hose available which are impregnated with antimicrobial agents which could be recommended) must be either decontaminated or destroyed. Any excessive sweating should be treated and skin care carefully monitored by Neil. It is often difficult for this sort of long-term personal care to be achieved and probably constitutes the biggest challenge for him. The podiatrist should approach this with understanding and good nature. It is imperative that the podiatrist develop a relationship with Neil within which Neil can admit to his failings and reaffirm an agreement to follow good health practice.

Chapter 23

The effect of the death
of a patient

*Bereavement is a darkness impenetrable to the imagination
of the unbereaved.*

Iris Murdoch

Ian Richards is a 50-year-old man who developed type 1 diabetes at the age
of 25. He was originally employed as a computer programmer and worked
within a team in a large corporate organisation. He was particularly adept
at his job and demonstrated not only good IT skills and knowledge but also
good interpersonal and management skills, which made him very popular
with his team. Ian's diabetes was particularly unstable, which resulted in
him having a lot of time off work; however, his employer was sympathetic
and supportive. In the past six months, Ian has been medically retired from
his position because of his diabetes and because of the associated medical
complications.

Ian is currently married to his second wife, Pamela, who is a 51-year-old
fit and a healthy, well-educated woman. Pamela was a primary school
teacher until recently; however, in the last two months she resigned from
her job to look after Ian. She does still do some supply teaching, as she still
likes to work and enjoys being with the children. However, her priority is her
husband and she always ensures that she can accompany him to the hospital
for his routine appointments. She has noticed that at home Ian is becoming
increasingly dependent upon her, which is cause for concern. This is also
Pamela's second marriage, in which she is very happy. Ian and Pamela have
children from their first marriages and also young grandchildren. They are
both doting and supportive grandparents.

Podiatric presentation

Ian presents with extensive foot ulceration, necrosis and osteomyelitis. He has become increasingly resistant to antibiotic therapy as a result of numerous infections and a deteriorating blood supply. He has recently been assessed by the vascular team, which has diagnosed peripheral neuropathy, vascular disease and renal failure. The digits on both the hands and feet have been affected and he has recently experienced necrosis of the smaller fingers.

Factors influencing Ian's behaviour

Ian has a familial history of diabetes, and, although disappointed that he developed the condition at a relatively young age, he was not surprised. In light of his condition, he has made deliberate choices about his health and has chosen not to drink alcohol or smoke cigarettes, which he believes will affect his diabetic control and prognosis. However, in recent years his diabetes has been increasingly unstable which has contributed to his current medical status.

Ian's wife is an optimistic enthusiastic person who on the whole believes that Ian will stabilise and be able to live a reasonable life. She has recently noted that there has been a decline of Ian's general state, which is causing her some concern. It has become evident that he is becoming physically weaker and that he is deteriorating more quickly than she had expected. She is very keen to be kept informed of what is happening and is active in trying to maintain his medical status. She tries to keep Ian busy and they play a lot of board games, such as Scrabble, together. However, just recently Ian has found difficulty in laying down the letter tiles because of the neuropathy in his fingers. He often drops the tiles, which he finds frustrating, particularly if it disrupts the board. They also enjoy completing crosswords and doing sudoku.

Challenge 1: Dealing with deteriorating health status

Pamela is finding it hard to come to terms with Ian's worsening state. She is hopeful that it is a temporary and that with the correct hospital treatment and support from her he will get better.

Denial is a common response to a stressful situation. It can be an important coping and defence mechanism. But it can delay the appropriate response to circumstances that require action and change. Pamela needs to be supported by the diabetes team and have the implications of Ian's situation realistically explained to her.

Diabetic nephropathy

Diabetic nephropathy is a clinical syndrome in people with diabetes. It is characterised by albuminuria occurring on at least two occasions separated by three to six months. Diabetic nephropathy is usually accompanied by hypertension, progressive rise in proteinuria and decline in renal function. In type 1 diabetes, five stages have been proposed (Fioretto *et al.*, 1992; Eknoyan *et al.*, 2003).

- Stages 1 and 2 are equivalent to *preclinical nephropathy*, and are only detected by imaging or biopsy.
- Stage 3, or *early nephropathy*. Early nephropathy presents as microalbuminuria, usually defined by an albuminuria level of 30–300 mg a day (or albumin/creatinine ratio of 30–300 mg/g [3.4–34.0 mg/mmol]).
- Stage 4 nephropathy is also known clinically as *late nephropathy*. Late nephropathy presents as macroalbuminuria, characterised by albuminuria greater than 300 mg a day (or albumin/creatinine ratio > 300 mg/g [34 mg/mmol]).
- Stage 5 represents the progression to *end stage renal disease.*

The cumulative risk of proteinuria rises 27–28% after 20 years of type 1 or type 2 diabetes. The overall prevalence of microalbuminuria and macroalbuminuria is 30–35% (Parving *et al.*, 2000).

Aetiology/risk factors

The risk factors of developing renal failure include: duration of diabetes, older age, male sex, smoking status and poor glycaemic control. These have all been found to be risk factors in the development of nephropathy (Ballard *et al.*, 1988; Marcantoni *et al.*, 1998). Moreover, certain ethnic groups seem to be at greater risk. African Americans, Native Americans and Mexican Americans have a much higher risk of developing end stage renal disease in the setting of diabetes compared with white people (Mokdad *et al.*, 2000; Molitch *et al.*, 2004). In the United States, African Americans with diabetes progress to end stage renal disease at a considerably more rapid rate than white people with diabetes do (Hsu *et al.*, 2003). In England, the rates for initiating treatment for end stage renal disease are 4.2 and 3.7 times higher for African Caribbeans and Indo-Asians respectively than for white people (Roderick *et al.*, 1996). Native Americans of the Pima tribe, in the south-west of the United States, have much higher rates of diabetic nephropathy than white people, and progress to end stage renal disease at a faster rate (Lemley, 2003).

Microalbuminuria is less pathognomonic of nephropathy among people with type 2 diabetes because hypertension, which is a common complication, can also cause microalbuminuria. Hypertension can also cause renal insufficiency; so, the time to development of renal insufficiency can be shorter in type 2 diabetes than in type 1. For people who have an atypical course, renal biopsy may be advisable. In addition, there are some differences in the progression of type 1 and type 2 diabetic nephropathy. In people with type 2 diabetes, albuminuria is more often present at diagnosis. Hypertension is more common in type 2 diabetic nephropathy. Finally, microalbuminuria is less predictive of late nephropathy in people with type 2 diabetes compared with type 1 (Powers, 2001).

Prognosis

People with microalbuminuria are at increased risk for progression to macroalbuminuria and end stage renal disease. The natural history of diabetic nephropathy is better defined in type 1 than type 2 diabetes. In type 2 diabetes, the course can be more difficult to predict, primarily because the date of onset of diabetes is less commonly known, and co-morbid conditions can contribute to renal disease. Without specific interventions, about 80% of people with type 1 diabetes, and 20–40% of people with type 2 diabetes with microalbuminuria, will progress to macroalbuminuria (Molitch, 2004). Diabetic nephropathy is associated with poor outcomes. In the United States, diabetes accounts for 48% of all new cases of end stage renal disease (US Renal Data System, 2000). In the United Kingdom, it is the most common cause of end stage renal disease, accounting for 20% of cases (Ansell and Feest, 2001). People with type 1 diabetes and proteinuria have been found to have a 40-fold greater risk of mortality than people without proteinuria have (Borch-Johnsen et al., 1985). The prognostic significance of proteinuria is less extreme in type 2 diabetes, although people with proteinuria have a fourfold risk of death compared with people without proteinuria (Mogensen, 1999). In addition, increased cardiovascular risk has been associated with albuminuria in people with diabetes (Mogensen, 1999).

Ian's deterioration

Ian suddenly deteriorated over a period of six months. He has become increasingly unable to stand and walk owing to bilateral muscle atrophy, which has resulted in him resorting to using a wheelchair. He has also found difficulty in getting out of bed without assistance and now relies on his wife for transfers. Ian has experienced numerous foot infections, which have been attended to by the podiatrist. However, these are taking considerably longer to heal, and once one has healed, another one appears.

Ian has also been diagnosed with a heart problem, which has resulted in him having a metallic heart valve fitted and the prescription of warfarin. He is beginning to develop heart failure, which is contributing to the development of necrotic leg ulcers and leg blisters. His wife recently noticed a pressure area developing over the sacral area and is concerned that it will ulcerate.

Ian has also reported that his eyesight does not appear to be as acute. After having his eyes tested, it appears that he has developed diabetic retinopathy.

Diabetic retinopathy is one of the most common causes of blindness in the United Kingdom. *Retinopathy* means damage to the capillaries that supply the retina, or the tissues in the back of the eye that deal with light. The damage to these vessels causes blood to leak. This can be a small leakage and confined to the retina, or it may be extensive and affect the vitreous gel that fills the main cavity of the eye, which can seriously affect vision.

Moreover, new, fragile blood vessels develop on the surface of the retina, particularly around the head of the optic nerve. The fragility of these vessels means that they can bleed easily. There are three main types of diabetic retinopathy:

- **Background retinopathy** is the least serious type of retinopathy. Small red dots will appear on your retina because of tiny swellings in the blood vessel walls. Proteins in the blood may also lead to small yellow patches developing on the back of the eye. This type of retinopathy does not require treatment but should be monitored by an ophthalmologist.
- **Pre-proliferative retinopathy** is when the retina swells and leaks blood which can start to obstruct vision, and reading small print may become particularly difficult. Laser treatment can be an option if leakage begins to threaten your vision. Laser treatment cannot restore any lost vision, but can be used to prevent further deterioration.
- **Proliferative retinopathy** rarely causes symptoms until it is too late. The symptoms include blurred vision and are likely to indicate that severe vitreous bleeding has developed, which will in turn usually cause a sudden loss of vision. Laser treatment is used to 'burn' the abnormal blood vessels to prevent further growth. The laser treatment does not target the blood vessels directly, but destroys those around your retina that have become starved of oxygen. The potential loss of sight is a further blow for Ian, both reducing his independence and increasing his depression.

Ian's dependence on Pamela has increased and she is now responsible for helping him to the toilet, completing hospital menu choices and feeding because of his loss of his digits and manual dexterity. She remains optimistic and believes that she is helping to improve his quality of life by providing nursing services that otherwise the nursing staff would have to provide. She believes that by undertaking these tasks the nursing staff can attend to other patients who are more in need than Ian is.

Pamela has spoken extensively with the diabetes team and so understands that Ian is seriously ill. She understands that he will probably not leave hospital but is resigned to this, and knows that for the foreseeable future her life will entail visiting and keeping Ian happy.

When admitted to hospital, Ian had extensive necrosis, foot ulceration and osteomyelitis. Osteomyelitis is an acute or chronic infection of the bone and bone marrow. Bone infection can be caused by bacteria, usually staphylococcus. In rare cases, it can be caused by fungus. Symptoms include pain and tenderness over the affected area of bone, and feeling unwell. It is a serious infection that needs prompt treatment with antibiotics. Surgery is usually needed if the infection becomes severe or persistent.

Unfortunately, Ian's infection has become antibiotic-resistant and his wounds are infected. Ian was referred to the vascular team, who advised a below-knee amputation. Pamela was extremely upset by this decision, but following advice from the surgeon felt that Ian had no other choice. Ian also believed it was the correct course of action and agreed to the surgery.

Unfortunately, Ian did not regain consciousness following the operation and remained in intensive care for 10 days. The prognosis for Ian was extremely poor and the palliative team was called to discuss the options for him with Pamela.

Pamela now understands that Ian is dying and she has to decide upon the best course of action for Ian, and for herself.

The palliative team has suggested that Ian be transferred to the local hospice, which would employ a *care for the dying pathway*. The pathway outlines the best plan of care for the dying person irrespective of their diagnosis. The dying process is unique to each person, but in the majority of cases a plan of care can be put into place to support the patient, hospital team and relatives or friends to achieve the best quality care at the end of life.

Care of the dying pathway

On commencing the pathway, the doctor or nurse will ask Pamela what she understands about Ian's condition and will give her the opportunity to ask any questions. The care for dying document acts as a guide for staff to clarify what Pamela knows and what she may need to know about the plan of care.

Pamela will provide her contact details, so that they can keep her informed of any change in Ian's condition.

Treatment/medication at the hospice

It may not be appropriate at this time to continue with tests, and more important that the staff talk about maintaining Ian's comfort, including discussions regarding position in bed and mouth care. The doctors will review the medication and stop any that is not helpful at this time.

Oxygen and fluid therapy will be reviewed and may be stopped if it were felt that they were not beneficial. New medication will be prescribed if new symptoms occur. It may not be possible to give medication by mouth at this time, so medication may be given by injection or sometimes, if necessary, by a continuous infusion by a small pump.

Religious, spiritual or cultural needs

The plan of care includes the need for staff to explore and meet the needs of Pamela and Ian with regard to their religious, spiritual or cultural needs. The services and support from the hospital chaplain will be offered. Not everyone who dies has a formal religion and the team will explore any other values, beliefs or cultural needs that Ian and Pamela may have at this time in order to meet their wishes.

Information and communication

Pamela will be given a leaflet that provides information on what to expect at this time in relation to any diminished need for food and drink, changes in breathing and withdrawing from the world.

The team looking after Ian will make regular assessments of his condition. Pamela will be encouraged to speak with the team regarding any worries or concerns that she may have.

Challenge 2: How can the podiatrist deal with the impact of death on family members?

Pamela feels that she should allow Ian to come home to die; however, she does not feel that she has the strength or ability to be able to look after him appropriately at home. She feels very upset about agreeing to have him transferred to the hospice but, conversely, does not feel that she could continue to live in the house if he were to die there.

Summary of important health psychology

The health psychology in this case involves both the patient and the carer. The origins of Pamela's denial should be carefully considered by the multidisciplinary team and handled with great sensitivity. Pamela may well be experiencing a period of anticipatory grief and be working her way through the accepted stages of grief. She should be enabled and supported through these difficult stages. Ian is coping by handing responsibility to the hospice and his medical team. This is an entirely understandable coping mechanism and should be considered as such. There are many, widely available, health psychology textbooks that examine coping strategies.

Implications for podiatric management

Management of Ian is multidisciplinary and multiprofessional. The role of the podiatrist is supportive and to offer palliative care. Of course, prevention of infection of ulceration is of paramount importance and extreme care must be taken when dealing with such vulnerable tissues. It must be remembered that the long-term care of patients such as Ian represent a huge challenge to the people who are working with them and their families. Arrangements for support and clinical supervision must be carefully considered. It is often the case that podiatrists find the inevitable end for these patients difficult. Colleagues should support each other through this period and should acknowledge the benefits that they did provide rather than dwelling on the negative aspects of the case.

Chapter 24

Challenging the current practice in podiatry

The worst loneliness is not to be comfortable with yourself.

Mark Twain

Sarah Terman is a 24-year-old single white woman who lives and works in a major city. She is employed as a full-time retail assistant in fashion, which she enjoys very much. She has been employed with this company since leaving college and wishes to pursue her career in the fashion industry. Her work requires her to spend most of the day on her feet. She is ambitious but has been unable to work for the last three weeks because of pain and swelling that she experiences in her heel and forefoot. This pain is becoming progressively worse.

Four years ago, Sarah acknowledged that she had pain in her feet. Initially, she tried to cope with the pain by using over-the-counter anti-inflammatory painkillers, which had little effect, and so she felt it necessary to see her GP because she was unable to work. In addition, she was not able to dress appropriately as she could not wear the 'nice' shoes. The GP diagnosed psoriatic arthritis. At first, she controlled her symptoms using the non-steroidal anti-inflammatory drug (NSAID) Naproxen, for what her GP thought might be caused by a Morton's Neuroma. This diagnosis was later discounted following an ultrasound scan. Over the next three months, Sarah exhibited signs and symptoms consistent with the development of an allergy to NSAIDs, and at the same time there was a marked deterioration in her pre-existing psoriasis. It was at this point that she was referred to the rheumatology department at her local hospital, where the consultant rheumatologist subsequently diagnosed her condition as psoriatic arthritis. Over the past three years, it has been difficult to achieve control of her symptoms with any consistency. Sarah has tried two disease-modifying anti-rheumatic drugs (DMARDs), which proved to be ineffective, and currently takes methotrexate. She still experiences flares of her arthritis and is being considered for one of the newer drugs, such as anti-TNFα therapy.

Factors influencing Sarah's behaviour

Having been referred to the podiatry clinic by the rheumatologist, at the first consultation Sarah explains, 'I'm afraid to say that I have the kind of feet that you would bury in the sand if you were on the beach. I can see from the expression on people's faces that I need to hide them.'

Sarah is experiencing difficulty in participating in the kind of social life that she desires. She is very self-conscious of the appearance of her feet and is unable to wear fashionable shoes. Her pain makes it impossible for her to go out with friends and the medication means that she has to be careful with her alcohol consumption. Moreover, the associated skin lesions are unsightly and prevent Sarah from wearing some of the clothes that she would like to.

The medication requires regular blood tests to monitor levels of liver and kidney function. Not only do these tests result in unsightly scars on her arms but also the necessity for them reinforces the fact that she has a chronic incurable disease at a relatively young age.

Presentation of psoriatic arthritis

Psoriatic arthritis is a chronic inflammatory arthritis with a heterogeneous presentation and varied clinical course. It can affect either gender at any age and the clinical features that characterise psoriatic arthritis include arthritis, tendonitis, enthesitis and dactylitis (inflammation and swelling of the digits). Characteristic psoriatic skin and nail lesions, or a history of such lesions, is also common. In addition to the dactylitis in this case, other common presentations in the feet include Achilles tendonitis and plantar fasciitis. There are also a number of clinical subgroups associated with psoriatic arthritis based on the clinical patterns of the disease. Management often requires shared care between the rheumatologist and the dermatologist in conjunction with the wider multidisciplinary team. Developments in pharmacological management such as including the use of biological agents have a role in the management of psoriatic arthritis.

Challenge 1: Given Sarah's characteristics, what particular difficulties could be encountered during the course of podiatric consultation?

There is an accepted understanding that inflammatory arthropathies such as psoriatic arthritis are associated with an increased frequency of disability, extra-articular co-morbidities, reduced quality of life and associated psychological impacts. Therefore, the condition impacts not only on sufferers' daily lives in terms of pain and disability but also on their relationships, social identity and sense of self (Nettleton, 2006). Indeed, Charmaz (2000) argues that these issues are as problematic in the social context as symptoms are in the medical context. The negative perceptions associated with chronic disease on both the physical body and its associated body image can be further reinforced by society's reactions to the appearance of the disease.

In Western culture in particular, there is a preoccupation with physical appearance, which is not only based upon but also constantly compared to unrealistically idealised images portrayed by the diet, fashion and advertising industries (Lonsdale, 1990; Caddick, 1995). This may lead to the development of a negative self-image for people with conditions such as psoriasis, which Murphy (1999) argues can lead to social isolation. This may be because of a tendency to avoid social situations owing to either a fear of embarrassment or a sense of guilt or shame. Both or either may occur in those with chronic illness, who may see themselves as not being able to cope in such situations (Murphy, 1999; Charmaz, 2000). Public reactions to disfiguring illness may vary. For instance, visible disability, such as hand deformity, may lead to sympathetic questions or expressions of empathy. By contrast, less invisible disabilities, as in the case of the feet, may lead to friends or family failing to acknowledge the true extent of pain and suffering. Such concern may be particularly important for adolescents and young adults, for whom acceptance into a peer group is especially important. In her autobiography as a young adult with rheumatoid arthritis, Peterson (2001) writes, 'I feel like Cinderella's ugly sister as I try to squash my feet into trainers.'

This further affects those with chronic disease by magnifying their sense of loss (Charmaz, 2000). Murphy (1999) writes that those who are disabled 'enter the social arena with a skewed perspective, not only are their bodies altered but ways of thinking about themselves have been transformed'.

There is a growing body of literature (Bassuk et al., 1999; Mendes de Leon et al., 1999; Berkman, 2005; Boden-Albala et al., 2005; Glass et al., 2006; Loucks et al., 2006) which highlights the importance of social interaction and engagement to human well-being. These are areas that often require adequate mobility and self-esteem in order to engage fully.

Social interactions are increasingly seen as key factors for maintaining psychosocial health in people who suffer from a range of chronic physical conditions. The impact of physical disability on social engagement cannot be denied. The Western medical model often fails to take account of the socially constructed realities of those living with chronic disease.

Challenge 2: What will be the likely effect of Sarah's condition on her social well-being?

Social contacts are of great importance for all of us. Foot complaints can make this valuable aspect of daily life particularly difficult for people with inflammatory arthritis. Some recreational activities allow opportunities for socialisation, and this in turn permits opportunities for the emotional benefits of socially acceptable touch, which, importantly in this context, are divorced from dependency on others for personal care needs (Young and Dinan, 2005). The ability to participate in low-impact aerobic exercise has been shown to have beneficial effects on more traditionally measured outcomes, such as walking time and grip strength (Neuberger *et al.*, 2007).

A further consideration is the recognition that some aspects of work require high levels of foot function, for example commuting by public transport, which may not be possible for those with considerable foot pain and may lead to early unemployment. Moreover, work roles can provide independence, and achievement makes a profound contribution to self-esteem. Thus, loss of employment has a profoundly negative impact in this respect (Abraído-Lanza and Revenson, 2006). Normal activities then require a conscious effort, which can be tiring and/or frustrating, and the effort required may not seem worthwhile. These factors have serious implications for psychological well-being (Bury, 1982; Locker, 1983; Ahlmén *et al.*, 2005; Abraído-Lanza and Revenson, 2006) and emphasise the need to consider the broader consequences of foot complaints on patients' everyday lives.

The loss of mobility, the inability to participate in valued life activities and reduced social interaction owing to foot pathology may also contribute to a range of co-morbidities. For example, if patients' mobility is limited and their function is impaired owing to foot involvement, they are less likely to participate in social and leisure activities that may confer a protective effect against cardiovascular disease. The significant contribution of social networks to cardiovascular disease prevention are well documented (Berkman and Syme, 1979).

Social interactions are rarely considered in existing treatment outcome measures, particularly those specific to foot complaints. This is possibly a reflection of the preoccupation of the medical model with alleviating symptoms and maintaining functional status (Evers *et al.*, 1998) and of the use of traditional measures of functional capacity (Neugebauer and Katz, 2004). It will prove useful to consider the fulfilment of social activities as an integral part of treatment planning, especially in light of the emphasis on patient-centred approaches highlighted in recent policy documents, including the Darzi review (Department of Health 2005a, 2005b, 2008).

It is important that the podiatrist consider the patient's social well-being and include this as a routine part of history-taking. The degree of social disability reported, compared to the desired level of activity, is a valid and reliable indicator of overall health status.

Summary of important health psychology

Social identity is a powerful influence on Sarah's behaviour. The concept of *identity* was originally introduced into the social sciences many years ago by Erikson (1950, 1968), who used the psychoanalytic term *ego identity*. Two themes have been distinguished in Erikson's original formulation (Gurin and Markus, 1990). The first is the individual's persistent sense of an enduring self across the lifespan, that is as they get older. The second is the continuous sense of sharing significant characteristics with other people who are both similar to us and important to us. This approach views individuals' identities as being formed, at least in part, in terms of the groups of which they are members (Duveen and Lloyd, 1986).

Individuals' social identities are constructed from the social representations of the significant groups in the society to which they belong. The development of social identities depends upon the internalisation of the social representations of these groups. In this context, the psychologist Moscovici introduced the term *social representation*. Social representations are the products or features of social groups and form organised systems of 'values, ideas and practices' (Moscovici, 1973). It is through access to shared social representations that individuals are able to understand the structure of their social lives and to interact with other people. The influence of social representations on individuals takes different forms (Duveen and Lloyd, 1990). Some social representations *require* individuals to adopt a particular social identity. This is the case, for example, with representations of age, gender or ethnicity, where individuals are generally constrained to construct prescribed social identities. In other instances, however, social representations require an individual who wishes to join a given social group to adopt a particular social identity. This may well include issues such as where and how people socialise, and their expectations of standards of dress.

Thus for Sarah, the inability to participate in the activities of her social group or to be fashionably attired may have deleterious effects upon her self-identity and thus her self-confidence and self-esteem. Therefore, her reduced choice in footwear may have unexpectedly far-reaching effects on Sarah's psychological well-being that might not be the case for other patients. The nature and extent of foot complaints leads to a series of difficulties for those with inflammatory arthropathies, including limitations of obligatory and, more importantly, valued life activities, a restricted choice of footwear, social isolation and reduced quality of life. In the busy clinical setting, it is all too easy to allow the assessment of foot complaints to be reduced to a mechanistic approach that leaves patients' feeling frustrated because they perceive that their concerns are deemed to be unimportant.

Implications for podiatric management

Foot complaints are common amongst those with psoriatic arthritis and the nature of this experience for many people with the disease is a multifaceted phenomenon. However, the assessment of foot complaints is often limited to measures of sensory characteristics rather than the maladaptive effects on social and occupational roles. The assessment of quality of life and valued life activities is also important, and is often under-represented in practice. A more in-depth understanding of the impact of social isolation and the need for social support for patients with foot complaints can provide insights into a more extensive range of interventions to complement current practice. This would not only improve our understanding of prognosis but also help to develop a more patient-centred approach to patient care.

Chapter 25

Coda

Rabbit is clever. Rabbit has Brain. I suppose that is why he never understands anything.

A. A. Milne

The scenarios described in this book have been carefully chosen in order to introduce the student to patients experiencing a range of life events. Appropriate psychological and sociological theory is provided and illustrated in the context of real patients from our combined clinical experience. In the early stages of a professional life, newly qualified practitioners may spend much of their time developing clinical skills in order to be able to cope with the demands of professional practice. At this stage, this book will help to explain some of the feelings that practitioners may experience.

A summary of the characters

The character of Jenny Fraser identifies some of issues associated with a new podiatry job. The early post-qualification period is a time when a range of skills are being developed, which are, for most newly qualified clinicians, skills that have not be encountered whilst being a student. The new clinician will be developing their time management skills and the general organisational skills required for running a busy clinic. In addition, the refinement of telephone, letter-writing and interpersonal skills will also become necessary, and can often be perceived as quite challenging. The combination of organisational problems such as insufficient back-up, waiting lists and the development of new skills can often lead to the experience of stress. The issues of work-related stress are considered in the case of Jenny Fraser. Strategies for maintaining a work–life balance are discussed.

Joseph Camilleri exemplifies the inseparability of national and religious culture from health-related behaviour. The difficulties of balancing religious and cultural influences are discussed. The impact of these influences on the podiatrist is discussed in detail. Attempts to change patient behaviour must be sensitive to such influences in order to be successful and ethically appropriate.

David Humphries, conversely, presents issues pertinent to practitioners who have been working in practice for some time. The need for continuous professional development and the mandatory requirement to demonstrate that such activities are taking place are discussed. The reaction and responses to such changes in practice by private practitioners are explored.

Suzi Dalton exhibits some of the problems that can be associated with middle age. In addition, she exemplifies some of the insecurities and vulnerability that are commonplace in contemporary British society.

Jayne Ellis portrays some of the frustrations experienced by senior podiatrists employed by large organisations. In addition, she has developed a work-related injury, which also contributes to her frustration.

Charles Walters and Dorothy Atkins are facing some of the challenges posed by the retirement years. Taken together, they provide a contrast which clearly demonstrates the crucial contribution that social support makes to health and well-being.

The aspirations and frustrations of a young executive are explored in the character of James Watt. James is a product of his times; he is competitive, materialistic and intolerant of having his chosen lifestyle frustrated.

Sensitivity to cultural differences is essential to podiatric practice, and the character of Sheetal Joshi explores this need in detail. The complications of language differences and working through interpreters are also considered.

Enid Hilton is experiencing bereavement. The processes she goes through as a result are an essential part of the understanding of all health care professionals, particularly those who deal predominantly with older people.

The influence of socio-economic status on health is illustrated in the case of Bill Canning. Bill is disempowered by his 'better off' peers, and his health-related behaviour is mediated by social exclusion.

People who suffer from severe mental health problems very commonly have difficulties with either drugs or alcohol. Such patients are often said to have a *dual diagnosis*, and have very complex needs, as is the case for Matthew Johnson.

Olivia Saunders presents an interesting challenge for the podiatrist, who is involved in a complex interaction involving a child and her parents.

The importance of confidentiality in professional practice is emphasised by the character of Peter Brennan, where the need to understand professional boundaries and competencies is explored in relation to his HIV status.

The ageing of the Western population is an issue of concern for health care providers, and older people represent the majority of patients in podiatric practice. Rose Stuart provides an example of an older person suffering from the early stages of dementia and demonstrates the need for professionals to consider not only the needs of their patients but also those of their patients' relatives and carers.

By contrast, Harriet Edmondson is a young woman who displays a number of the difficulties associated with adolescence. The impact of the life changes that early adulthood brings are a profound influence on her behaviour.

Homelessness among the UK population has increased markedly in the last few decades, and homeless people are particularly vulnerable to a range of risks and illnesses less often found in more fortunate members of society. The needs of homeless people are complex and there is a common tendency for statutory services to be inadequate to meet them in an integrated way. Some of the associated problems are discussed in the chapter concerning John Piper.

Margaret Knowles, like all of the characters in this book, is based on a real person. Her story clearly portrays the compromises that people are prepared to endure in order to meet the needs of others above those of themselves. In Margaret's case, her attachment to her family was overwhelmingly more important to her than her own welfare, with tragic consequences.

Sophie Miller is an adolescent who suffers from a serious physical disability. She is disillusioned with conventional medicine and seeks alternatives. She is not understood by her family, who are unable to support her.

The character of George Archer is used to illustrate current psychological theory in relation to decision-making processes and substance use. George is used to explain why people find giving up addictive behaviours so difficult and provides a theoretical model through which this is explained.

Neil Anderson is an interesting character who will pose a challenge to the podiatrist. For Neil, the needs of others are more important than his own well-being. The dilemma presented to the podiatrist is carefully considered and strategies are provided to enable the clinician to cope with such issues.

The character of Ian Richards is presented to explore the complex issues of working with chronically ill patients, and the possible outcomes that arise from such conditions.

The final character, Sarah Terman, presents to the podiatrist challenges and frustrations of being a relatively young person coping with a chronic long-term debilitating condition. The chapter contextualises the issues that are pertinent to such patients.

Psychological theory and its application to clinical practice

Clearly, as the podiatrist's clinical and life experience expands, so too will his/her abilities and confidence to work with a wide range of patients grow. Developing an understanding of psychosocial issues in relation to patients will not only improve the care that he/she can offer but will also result in a more rewarding and satisfying career. This aspect of professional practice will continue to grow long after the podiatrist's clinical skills have reached a point of excellence.

The psychological theory expounded in this book will serve as an aid to your clinical practice. Understanding the principles outlined in each chapter will help you to deal more effectively with a wide range of patients and their problems. Podiatry and physiotherapy students spend three years developing their intellectual abilities in terms of diagnosis, clinical reasoning and treatment planning. Equally important, in our view, is the need for students to develop what has become known as *emotional intelligence*. Emotional intelligence involves the ability to be sensitive to the emotions and reactions of others. It also involves understanding one's own emotional reactions to the behaviour of other people in general. In the case of clinicians, this particularly applies to their interactions with patients. A number of processes have been identified which, taken together, provide a measure of individuals' emotional intelligence. First, the ability to interpret other people's emotions as expressed in their facial expressions, body language, general demeanour and tone of voice, rather than overtly verbally. This ability represents emotional intelligence of the most basic kind. Second, emotional intelligence involves an ability to employ one's thought processes in relation to changing mood states that are appropriate to the task being undertaken. Third, emotional intelligence requires an ability to understand the language of emotional experience and to appreciate that complex relationships occur in which conflicting emotions may interact and how other people's emotions may change over time in relation to their circumstances. Finally, emotionally intelligent people are able to control their own emotional responses in order to achieve their intended goals. This last ability is of critical importance among health professionals; patients can be demanding, frustrating and irritating and the reactions that these characteristics can invoke in their therapists may not always be conducive to a therapeutic relationship.

A detailed theoretical consideration of emotional intelligence, its nature and measurement are beyond the scope of this book; however, it is provided extensively elsewhere (Goleman, 1995).

However, no amount of theorising can substitute for important qualities, which the reader must learn to develop for themselves. Warmth, empathy and human understanding cannot be taught solely in a classroom, seminar or by reading a book. They are, however, the very attributes that will distinguish an adequate technician from a true practitioner.

References

Abbott, A. (1981) Status and status strain in the professions. *American Journal of Sociology*, **86** (4), 819–835.

Abraído-Lanza, A.F., Revenson, T.A. (2006) Illness intrusion and psychological adjustment to rheumatic diseases: A social identity framework. *Arthritis Care and Research*, **55** (2), 224–232.

Ahlmén, M., Nordenskiöld, U., Archenholtz, B. *et al.* (2005) Rheumatology outcomes: The patient's perspective: A multicentre focus group interview study of Swedish rheumatoid arthritis patients. *Rheumatology*, **44** (1), 105–110.

Aidman, E.V., Woollard, S. (2003) The influence of self-reported exercise addiction on acute emotional and physiological responses to brief exercise deprivation. *Psychology of Sport and Exercise*, **3** (4), 225–236.

Ajzen, I., Madden, T.J. (1986) Prediction of goal-directed behaviour: Attitudes intentions, and perceived behavioral control. *Journal of Experimental Social Psychology*, **22** (4), 453–474.

Alder, B. (1999) *Psychology of Health: Applications of Health Psychology for Health Professionals*, (2nd edn.). Harwood Academic Pubs, Amsterdam.

Altman, D.G., Levine, D.W., Coeytaux, R., Slade, J., Jaffe, R. (1996) Tobacco promotion and susceptibility to tobacco use among adolescents aged 12 through 17 years in a nationally representative sample. *American Journal of Public Health*, **86** (11), 1590–1593.

American Psychological Association (2006) Research shows how religious belies can protect psychological well-being during stressful experiences. http://www.apa.org/releases/religious06.html, accessed 11 May 2008.

Andreasen, N.C., Arndt, S., Alliger, R., Miller, D., Flaum, M. (1995) Symptoms of schizophrenia: Methods, meanings, and mechanisms. *Archives of General Psychiatry*, **52** (5), 341–351.

Angell, M. (1991) The case of Helga Wanglie: A new kind of 'right to die' case. *New England Journal of Medicine*, **325**, 511–512.

Ansell, D., Feest, T. (2001) *UK Renal Registry Report*. UK Renal Registry, Bristol.

Antonovsky, A. (1979) *Health, Stress and Coping: New Perspectives on Mental and Physical Well-Being*. Jossey-Bass, San Francisco.

Argyle, M. (1990) *Bodily Communication*, (2nd edn.). Routledge, London.

Asch, S.E. (1946) Forming impressions of personality. *Journal of Abnormal and Social Psychology*, **41** (3), 258–290.

Bäckman, G. (1990) Life control and perceived health. *Tijdschr Soc Gezondheidsz*, Supp II, 123–127.

Bäckman, G. (1991) Livskontroll: en buffert mot ohalsa? (Life control: a buffer against ill health?) In: *Etik, Solidaritet, Valfard: Festskrift till Harald Swender (Ethics, Solidarity, Welfare: Festschrift for Harald Swedner)*, (eds B. Bergsten, A. Bjerkmans, H.E. Hermansssohn, J. Israel). Diadalos, Uddevalla, Sweden.

Ballard, D.J., Humphrey, L.L., Melton, L.J. *et al.* (1988) Epidemiology of persistent proteinuria in type II diabetes mellitus: Population-based study in Rochester, Minnesota. *Diabetes*, **37**, 405–412.

Bandura, A. (1973) *Aggression: A Social Learning Analysis*. Prentice Hall, Englewood Cliffs, NJ.

Bandura, A. (1977) Self efficacy: Towards a unifying theory of behavioural change. *Psychological Review*, **84** (2), 191–215.

Barrow, S.M., Herman, D.B., Cordova, P., Streuning, E.L. (1999) Mortality among homeless shelter residents in New York City. *American Journal of Public Health*, **89** (4), 529–534.

Bassuk, S.S., Glass, T.A., Berkman, L.F. (1999) Social disengagement and incident cognitive decline in community-dwelling elderly persons. *Annals of Internal Medicine*, **131** (3), 165–173.

Beale, N. (2001) Unequal to the task: Deprivation, health and UK general practice at the millennium. *British Journal of General Practice*, **51** (467), 478–485.

Becker, H.S., Geer, B., Hughes, E.C., Strauss, A.L. (1961) *Boys in White*. Chicago University Press.

Becker, M.H., Rosenstock, I.M. (1984) Compliance with medical advice. In: *Healthcare and Human Behaviour*, (eds A. Steptoe, A. Mathews). Academic Press, London.

Beecher, H.K. (1956) Relationship of significance of wound to pain experienced. *Journal of the American Medical Association*, **161**, 1609–1613.

Benjaminsen, S., Krarup, G., Lauritsen, R. (1990) Personality, parental rearing behaviour and parental loss in attempted suicide: A comparative study. *Acta Psychiatrica Scandinavica*, **82** (5), 389–397.

Berkman, L.F. (2005) Tracking social and biological experiences: Circulation. *Journal of the American Heart Association*, **111** (23), 3022–3024.

Berkman, L.F., Syme, S.L. (1979) Social networks, host resistance and mortality: A nine year follow up study of Alameda county residents. *American Journal of Epidemiology*, **109** (2), 186–204.

Berkman, L.F, Glass, T., Brissette, I., Seeman, T.E. (2000) From social integration to health: Durkheim in the new millennium. *Social Science & Medicine*, **51** (6), 843–857.

Berkowitz, A. (1993) *Aggression: Its Causes, Consequences and Control*. McGraw-Hill, New York.

Billings, J.S. (1891) Vital statistics of the Jews. *New American Review*, **153**, 70–84.

Birtles, M., Leah, C. (2006) *Musculoskeletal Disorders in Podiatry & Chiropody Professionals*, Health & Safety Laboratory, London, http://www.hse.gov.uk/research/hsl_pdf/2006/hsl0660.pdf, accessed 20 February 2009.

Bjorkqvist, K., Lagerspetz, K.M.J., Kaukiainen, A. (1992) Do girls manipulate and boys fight? Developmental trends regarding direct and indirect aggression. *Aggressive Behaviour*, **18**, 157–166.

Blakeslee, T.J., Morris, J.L. (1987) Cuboid syndrome and the significance of midtarsal joint stability. *Journal of the American Podiatric Medical Association*, **777** (12), 638–642.

Boden-Albala, B., Litwak, P.H.E., Elkind, V., Rundek, T., Sacco, R.L. (2005) Social isolation and outcomes post stroke. *Neurology*, **64** (11), 1888–1892.

Bond, J., Bond, S. (1994) *Sociology and Health Care: An introduction for nurses and other health care professionals*, (2nd edn.). Churchill Livingstone, Edinburgh.

Bond, J., Coleman, P. (eds) (1990) *Ageing in Society: An introduction to Social Gerontology*. Sage, London.

Borch-Johnsen, K., Andersen, P.K., Deckert, T. (1985) The effect of proteinuria on relative mortality in type 1 (insulin-dependent) diabetes mellitus. *Diabetologia*, **28**, 590–596.

Borthwick, A.M. (2000) Challenging medicine: The case of podiatric surgery: Work, employment and society. *British Journal of Podiatry*, **14** (2), 369–383.

Bowlby, J. (1969, 1973, 1980) *Attachment and Loss: Volumes 1–3*. Basic Books, New York.

Breakey, J.W. (1997) Body image: the inner mirror. *Journal of Prosthetics and Orthotics*, **9** (3), 107–112.

British Heart Foundation Statistics (2000) *Coronary Heart Disease Statistics: British Heart Foundation statistics database annual compendium*. Department of Public Health, University of Oxford, Oxford.

Brody, H. (1985) Autonomy revisited: Progress in medical ethics: Discussion paper. *Journal of the Royal Society of Medicine*, **78** (5), 380–387.

Burke, P.J. (1991) Identity, processes and social stress. *American Sociological Review*, **56** (6), 836–49.

Bury, M. (1982) Chronic illness as biographical disruption. *Sociology of Health and Illness*, **4** (2), 167–182.

Byrd, R.C. (1988) Positive therapeutic effects of intercessory prayer in a coronary care unit population. *Southern Medical Journal*, **81** (7), 826–829.

Caddick, A. (1995) Making babies, making sense: Reproductive technologies, postmodernity, and the ambiguities of feminism. In: *Troubled Politics: Critical Perspectives on Postmodernism, Medical Ethics, and the Body*, (ed. Paul A. Komesaroff). Duke University Press, Durham, NC.

Calvin, R.L, Lane, P.L. (1999) Perioperative uncertainty and state anxiety of orthopaedic surgical patients. *Orthopaedic Nursing*, **18** (6), 61–6.

Cameron, L., Leventhal, E.A., Leventhal, H. (1995) Seeking medical care in response to symptoms and life stress. *Psychosomatic Medicine*, **57** (1), 37–47.

Carayon, P., Smith, M.J., Haims, M.C. (1999) Work, organisation, job stress and work related musculoskeletal disorders. *Human Factors*, **41** (4), 644–663.

Carr-Saunders, A.P., Wilson, P.A. (1933) *The Professions*. Oxford University Press.

Cast, A., Burke, P. (2002) A theory of self esteem. *The University of North Carolina Press*, **80** (3), 1041–1068.

Chapman, C., Kishore, A. (1999) Information needs and anxiety in patients anticipating toe nail surgery. *British Journal of Podiatry*, **2** (4), 108–118.

Chapman, C.L., De Castro, J.M. (1990) Running addiction: Measurement and associated psychological characteristics. *Journal of Sports Medicine & Physical Fitness*, **30** (3), 283–90.

Charmaz, K. (2000) Experiencing chronic illness. In: *Handbook of Social Studies in Health and Medicine*, (eds G.L. Albrecht, R. Fitzpatrick, S.C. Scrimshaw). Sage, London.

Cheung, A.M., Hwang, S.W. (2004) Risk of death among homeless women: A cohort study and review of the literature. *Canadian Medical Association Journal*, **170** (8), 1243–1247.

Chrousos, G.P., Gold, P.W. (1992) The concepts of stress and stress disorders: Overview of physical and behavioural homeostasis. *Journal of the American Medical Association*, **267** (9), 1244–1252.

Colliver, J.A. (2000) Effectiveness of problem-based learning curricula: Research and theory. *Academic Medicine*, **75** (3), 259–266.

Colyer, H. (2004) The construction and development of health professions: Where will it end? *Journal of Advanced Nursing*, **48** (4), 406–412.

Comstock, G.W., Partridge, K.B. (1972) Church attendance and health. *Journal of Chronic Diseases*, **25** (12), 665–672.

Concha, J.M., Moore, L.S., Holloway, W.J. (1998) Antifungal activity of Melaleuca Alternifolia (tea tree oil) against various pathogenic organisms. *Journal of the American Podiatry Association*, **88** (10), 489–492.

Cote, M. (1993) Case method case teaching and the making of a manager. In: *Case Method and Application: Innovation Through Co-operation*, (ed. H.E. Klein). World Association for Case Method Research and Application, Needham, MA.

Cox, T. (1978) *Stress*. Macmillan Press, London.

Dahlin, L., Cederblad, M., Antonovsky, A., Hagnell, O. (1990) Childhood vulnerability and adult invincibility. *Acta Psychiatrica Scandinavica*, **82** (3), 228–232.

Davis, C., Katzman, D.K., Kirsh, C. (1999) Compulsive physical activity in adolescents with anorexia nervosa: A psychobehavioral spiral of pathology. *Journal of Nervous and Mental Diseases*, **187** (6), 336–342.

Delisle, A.M. (1998) What does solitude mean to the aged? *Canadian Journal of Aging*, **7** (4), 358–371.

Department of Health (2000) *The NHS Plan*. HMSO, London.

Department of Health (2005a) *'Now I feel tall': What a patient-led NHS feels like*. HMSO, London.

Department of Health (2005b) *Creating a Patient-led NHS*. HMSO, London.

Department of Health (2008) *High Quality Care for All*. HMSO, London.

Devereux, J.J., Buckle, P.W., Vlachonikolis, I.G. (1999) Interactions between physical and psychological risks factors at work increase the risk of back disorders: An epidemiological approach. *Occupational Environmental Medicine*, **56** (5), 343–353.

Diabetes UK (2006) *The National Minimum Skills Framework for Commissioning of Foot Care Services for People with Diabetes*. Foot in Diabetes UK, Diabetes UK, The Association of British Clinical Diabetologists, The Primary Care Diabetes Society and The Society of Chiropodists and Podiatrists, London, http://www.feetforlife.org/download/4033/NatMinSkillFramewkFootNov06.pdf, accessed 25 February 2009.

Dickson, D.A., Hargie, O., Morrow, N.C. (1997) *Communication Skills Training for Health Professionals: An instructor's handbook*, (2nd edn.). Chapman & Hall, London.

Diedrick, P. (1991) Comparison of gender differences. In: *Women and Divorce/Men and Divorce: Gender Differences in Separation, Divorce and Remarriage*, (ed. S. Volgy). Haworth Press, New York.

Dixon, L. (1999) Dual diagnosis of substance abuse in schizophrenia: Prevalence and impact on outcomes. *Schizophrenia Research*, **35** (suppl. 1), S93–S100.

Donaldson, C. (1999) Valuing the benefits of publicly-provided health care: Does 'ability to pay' preclude the use of willingness? *Social Science & Medicine*, **49** (4), 551–563.

Donaldson, M.S., Yordy, K.D., Lohr, K.N., Vanselow, N. (eds) (1996) *Primary Care: America's Health in a New Era*. National Academy Press, Washington.

Dowrenwend, B., Pearlin, L., Clayton, P. *et al.* (1982) Report on stress and life events. In: *Stress and Human Health: Analysis and implications of research*, (eds G.R. Elliott, C. Eisdorfer). Springer, New York.

Dunn, D.S. (1996) Well being following amputation: Salutary effects of positive meaning, optimism, and control. *Rehabilitation Psychology*, **41** (4), 285–302.

Dunn, J.R., Hayes, M.V. (2000) Social inequality, population health and housing: A study of two Vancouver neighbourhoods. *Social Science & Medicine*, **51** (4), 563–587.

Durkheim, E. (1897) *Le Suicide*. Felix Alcan, Paris.

Duveen, G.M., Lloyd, B.B. (1986) The significance of social identities. *British Journal of Social Psychology*, **25**, 219–230 and 235–236.

Duveen, G.M., Lloyd, B.B. (eds) (1990) *Social Representations and the Development of Knowledge*. Cambridge University Press.

Ecob, R., Davey Smith, G. (1999) Income and health: What is the nature of the relationship? *Social Science & Medicine*, **48** (5), 693–705.

Eknoyan, G., Hostetter, T., Bakris, G.L. *et al.* (2003) Proteinuria and other markers of chronic kidney disease: A position statement of the National Kidney Foundation (NKF) and the National Institute of Diabetes and Digestive and Kidney Diseases (NIDDK). *American Journal of Kidney Disease*, **42** (4), 617–622.

Elton, M.A. (1977) Medical autonomy, challenge and response. In: *Conflicts in the National Health Service*, (eds K. Bernard, K. Lee). Croom Helm, London.

Enas, E.A., Dhawan, J., Petkar, S. (1997) Coronary artery disease in Asian Indians: Lessons learnt and the role of lipoprotein. *Indian Heart Journal*, **49** (11), 25–34.

Enas, E.A., Yusuf, S., Mehta, J. (1996) Coronary artery disease in South Asians: Meeting of the International Working Group. *Indian Heart Journal*, **48**, 727–732.

Erikson, E.H. (1950) *Childhood and Society*. Norton, New York.

Erikson, E.H. (1968) *Identity, Youth and Crisis*. Norton, New York.

Evers, A.W.M., Taal, E., Kraaimaat, F.W. *et al.* (1998) A comparison of two recently developed health status instruments for patients with arthritis: Dutch–AIMS2 and IRGL. *British Journal of Rheumatology*, **37** (2), 157–164.

Farkas, A.J., Pierce, J.P., Zhu, S.-H. *et al.* (1996) Addiction versus stages of change models in predicting smoking cessation. *Addiction*, **91** (9), 1271–1280.

Farndon, L., Vernon, W., Potter, J. (2002) The professional role of the podiatrist in the new millennium: An analysis of current practice. Paper 1. *British Journal of Podiatry*, **5** (3), 68–72.

Fioretto, P., Steffes, M.W., Brown, D.M., Mauer, S.M. (1992) An overview of renal pathology in insulin-dependent diabetes mellitus in relationship to altered glomerular hemodynamics. *American Journal of Kidney Disease*, **20** (6), 549–558.

Fishbein, M., Ajzen, I. (1975) *Belief, Attitudes, Intentions and Behavior: An introduction to theory and research*. Addison-Wesley, Los Angeles.

Fisher, B., Neve, H., Heritage, Z. (1999) Community development, user involvement, and primary health care. *British Medical Journal*, **318** (7186), 749–750.

Fisher, S. (1973) *Body Consciousness*. Open Forum, London.

Formosa, C. (2008) Culture and the management of diabetes in Malta. PhD thesis, University of Brighton.

Freidson, E. (1970) *Profession of Medicine*. Dodd Mead & Co., New York.

Friedman, M., Rosenman, R.H. (1974) *Type A Behaviour and Your Heart*. Knopf, New York.

Friedson, E. (1971) *The Professions and Their Prospects*. Sage, London.

Fulder, S., Munro, R. (1985) Complementary medicine in the United Kingdom: Patients, practitioners and consultants. *The Lancet*, **2** (8454), 542–545.

Gafaranga, J., Britten, N. (2003) 'Fire away': The opening sequence in general practice consultations. *Family Practice*, **20** (3), 242–247.

Garcia, M.J., McNamara, P.M., Gordon, T., Kannell, W.B. (1974) Morbidity and mortality in diabetics in the Framingham population: Sixteen year follow-up. *Diabetes*, **23** (2), 105–111.

Gergen, K.J. (1997) Social psychology as social construction: The emerging vision. In: *The Message of Social Psychology*, (eds C. McGarty, A. Haslam). Blackwell, Oxford.

Glass, T.A., De Leon, C.F., Bassuk, S.S., Berkman, L.F. (2006) Social engagement and depressive symptoms in later life: Longitudinal findings. *Journal of Aging and Health*, **18** (4), 604–628.

Goleman, D. (1995) *Emotional Intelligence*. Bantam Books, New York.

Golomer, E., Chatellier, K. (1990) Anthropométrie du pied du chausson de pointe et pathologie cutanée. *Cinesiologie*, **29**, 277–282.

Greenwood, E. (1957) Attributes of a profession. *Social Work*, **2** (3), 44–55.

Grembowski, D., Patrick, D., Diehr, P., Durham, M., Beresford, S., Kay, E. (1993) Self efficacy and health behaviour among older adults. *Journal of Health & Social Behaviour*, **34** (2), 89–104.

Grosarth-Maticek, R., Kanariz, D.T., Schmidt, P. (1982) Psychosomatic processes in the development of cancerogenesis. *Psychotherapy Psychosomatics*, **38**, 284–302.

Gunner, G., Knott, H. (1997) *Homelessness on Civvy Street*. Ex-Service Action Group, London.

Gurin, P., Markus, H. (1990) Cognitive consequences of gender identity. In: *The Social Identity of Women*, (eds S. Skiffington, D. Baker). Sage, London.

Habermas, J. (1989) *Theory of Communicative Action: Volume 2: Lifeworks and system: A critique of functionalist reason*. Beacon, Boston.

Hagberg, M., Morgenstern, H., Kelsh, M. (1992) Impact of occupations and job tasks on the prevalence of carpal tunnel syndrome. *Scandinavian Journal of Environment and Health*, **18** (6), 337–345.

Halford, V., Birch, I. (2005) The perceived causes of hand pain in podiatrists. *British Journal of Podiatry*, **8** (3), 102–107.

Halford, V., Cohen, H.H. (2003) Technology use and psychosocial factors in self reporting of musculoskeletal disorder symptoms in call centre workers. *Journal of Safety Research*, **34** (2), 167–73.

Hall, A., Wellman, B. (1985) Social networks and social support. In: *Social Support and Health*, (eds S. Cohen, S.L. Syme). Academic Press, Orlando, FL.

Hanson, B.S., Isacsson, S.O., Janzon, L., Lindell, S.E. (1990) Social support and quitting smoking for good: Is there an association? Results from the study 'Men born in 1914', Malmo, Sweden. *Addictive Behaviours*, **15** (3), 221–233.

Harter, S. (1985) Competence as a dimension of self-evaluation: Towards a comprehensive model of self worth. In: *The Development of the Self*, (ed. R.L. Leahy). Academic Press, Orlando, FL.

Harter, S. (1988a) The determinations and mediations of global self-worth in children. In: *Contemporary Topics in Developmental Psychology*, (ed. N. Eisberg). Wiley-Interscience, New York.

Harter, S. (1988b) Developmental processes in the construction of the self. In: *Integrative Processes and Socialism: Early to middle childhood*, (eds T.D. Yankey, J.E. Johnson). John Wiley & Sons, New York.

Hartup, W.W. (1996) Cooperation, close relationships and cognitive development. In: *The Company They Keep: Friendship in childhood and adolescence*, (eds W.M. Bukowski, A.F. Newcomb, W.W. Hartup). Cambridge University Press, New York.

Health and Safety Executive (2007) *HSE Statistics: Causes and kind of disease – Musculoskelatal Disorders*, http://www.hse.gov.uk/research/hsl_pdf/2006/hsl0660.pdf, accessed 26 February 2009.

Heider, F. (1958) *The Psychology of Interpersonal Relations*. John Wiley & Sons, New York.

Hill, A.B. (1965) The environment and disease: Association or causation? *Proceedings of the Royal Society of Medicine*, **58** (May), 1217–1219.

Hjortdahl, P., Laerum, E. (1992) Continuity of care in general practice: effect on patient satisfaction. *British Medical Journal*, **304**, 1287–1290.

Holahan, C., Holahan, C. (1987) Self-efficacy social support and depression in aging: A longitudinal analysis. *Journal of Gerontology*, **42** (1), 65–68.

Hsu, C.Y., Lin, F., Vittinghoff, E., Shlipak, M.G. (2003) Racial differences in the progression from chronic renal insufficiency to end-stage renal disease in the United States. *Journal of the American Society of Nephrology*, **14** (11), 2902–2907.

Hunter, D., Killoran, A. (2004) *Tackling Health Inequalities: Turning policy into practice?*, http://www.who.int/rpc/meetings/en/Hunter_Killoran_Report.pdf, accessed 16 February 2009.

Ikeda, J., Naworski, P. (1992) *Am I fat? Helping young children accept differences in body size*. ETR Associates, Santa Cruz, CA.

Ishorst-Witte, F., Heinemann, A., Puschel, K. (2001) Erkrankungen und Todesursachen bei Wohnungslosen. *Archives für Kriminologie*, **208** (5, 6), 129–138.

Israel, B.A., House, J.S., Schurman, S.J., Heaney, C., Mero, R.P. (1989) The relation of personal resources, participation, influence, interpersonal relationships and coping strategies to occupational stress, job strains and health: A multivariate analysis. *Work & Stress*, **3**, 163–194.

Jackson, S.E. (1983) Participation in decision making as a strategy for reducing job-related strain. *Journal of Applied Psychology*, **68**, 3–19.

James, C.W., McNeils, K.C., Cohen, D.M., Szabo, S., Bincsik, A.K. (2001) Recurrent ingrown toenails secondary to indinavir/ritonavir combination therapy. *Annals of Pharmacotherapy*, **35** (7), 881–884.

Jenkins, C.D. (1971) Psychologic and social precursors of coronary disease. *New England Journal of Medicine*, **284** (6), 244–255.

Johnston, M. (1996) Models of disability. *The Psychologist*, **9** (May), 205–210.

Jung, C.G. (1928, 1943) Two essays on analytical psychology. *The Collected Works*, **7**, 188–211.

Kalimo, R., Vuori, J. (1990) Work and sense of coherence: Resources for competence and life satisfaction. *Behavioural Medicine*, **16** (2), 76–89.

Kalimo, R., Vuori, J. (1991) Work factors and health: The predictive role of pre-employment experiences. *Journal of Occupational Psychology*, **64** (2), 97–115.

Kaplan, S.H., Greenfield, S., Ware, J.E., Jr. (1989) Assessing the effects of physician–patient interactions on the outcomes of chronic disease. *Medical Care*, **27** (3) (suppl.), S110–S127.

Karseras, P., Hopkins, E. (1987) *British Asians' Health in the Community*. John Wiley & Sons, Chichester.

Kasl, S.A., Cobb, S. (1966) Health behaviour and illness behaviour and sick role behaviour. *Archives of Environmental Health*, **12**, 246–266.

Kawachi, I., Kennedy, B.P., Lochner, K., Prothrow-Stith, D. (1997) Social capital, income inequality and mortality. *American Journal of Public Health*, **87** (9), 1491–1498.

Khan, M.T. (2000a) Clinical evaluation of homeopathic podiatry in the treatment of diabetic foot ulcers. *British Homoeopathic Journal*, **89** (suppl. 1), S67.

Khan, M.T. (2000b) Clinical application of homeopathic podiatry as used at The Royal London Homeopathic Hospital (RLHH). *British Homoeopathic Journal*, **89** (suppl. 1), S53.

King, H., Locke, F.B. (1980) American White Protestant Clergy as a low risk population for mortality research. *Journal of the National Cancer Institute*, **65** (5), 1115–1124.

Kirsch, I., Sapirstein, G. (1998) Listening to Prozac but hearing placebo: A meta-analysis of antidepressant medication. *Prevention & Treatment*, **1** (2), ArtID 2a.

Koenig, H.G. (1998) Religious attitudes and practices of hospitalized medically ill older adults. *International Journal of Geriatric Psychiatry*, **13** (4), 213–224.

Koenig, H.G., George, L.K., Hays, J.C., Larson, D.B., Cohen, H.J., Blazer, D.G. (1998) The relationship between religious activities and blood pressure in older adults. *International Journal of Psychiatry in Medicine*, **28** (2), 189–213.

Kohler, C.G., Moberg Gur, P.J., O'Connor, R.E., Sperling, M., Doty, M.R., Richard, L. (2001) Olfactory dysfunction in schizophrenia and temporal lobe epilepsy neuropsychiatry. *Neuropsychology & Behavioral Neurology*, **14** (2), 83–88.

Kübler-Ross, E. (1969) *On Death and Dying*. Tavistock, New York.

Larson, M. (1977) *The Rise of Professionalism*. University of California Press.

Layzell, P. (2004) Out on a limb: Work related upper limb disorders in podiatrists. *Podiatry Now*, **7** (1), 14–17.

Lazarus, R. (1991) Psychological stress in the workplace. *Journal of Social Behavior and Personality*, **6** (7), 1–13.

Lazarus, R.S. (1966) *Psychological Stress and the Coping Process*. McGraw-Hill, New York.

Le Grand, J. (1993) Equity in the distribution of healthcare: The British debate. In: *Equity in the Finance and Delivery of Healthcare: An international perspective*, (eds A. Wagstaff, F. Rutten, E.K.A.V. Doorslaer). Oxford University Press.

Lee, R.T., Ashforth, B.E. (1996) A meta analytic examination of the correlates of the three dimensions of job burnout. *Journal of Applied Psychology* **81** (2), 123–133.

Lemley, K.V. (2003) A basis for accelerated progression of diabetic nephropathy in Pima Indians. *Kidney International*, (suppl.), S38–S42.

Leopold, N., Cooper, J., Clancy, C. (1996) Sustained partnership in primary care. *Journal of Family Practice*, **42** (2), 129–37.

Levenson, H. (1981) Differentiating among internality powerful others and chance. In: *Research with the Locus of Control Construct: Volume 1*, (ed. H.M. Lefcourt). Academic Press, New York.

Leventhal, H., Benyamini, Y. (1997) Lay beliefs about health and illness. In: *Cambridge Handbook of Psychology Health and Medicine*, (eds A. Baum, S. Newman, J. Weinman, R. West, M. McManus). Cambridge University Press.

Levin, J.S. (1994) Religion and health: Is there an association, is it valid, and is it causal? *Social Science and Medicine*, **38** (11), 1475–1482.

Levin, J.S., Schiller, P.L. (1987) Is there a religious factor in health? *Journal of Religion and Health*, **26**, 9–36.

Levin, J.S., Vanderpool, H.Y. (1989) Is frequent religious attendance really conducive to better health? Towards an epidemiology of religion. *Social Science and Medicine*, **24**, 1475–1482.

Light, D., Jr. (1979) Uncertainty and control in professional training. *Journal of Health and Social Behavior*, **20** (4), 310–22.

Lindquist, C.A., Whitehead, J.T. (1986) Burnout, job stress and job satisfaction among southern correctional officers: Perceptions and casual factors. *Journal of Offender Counselling Services and Rehabilitation*, **10**, 5–26.

Locke, E.A. (1968) Toward a theory of task motivation and incentives. *Organisational Behaviour and Human Performance*, **3**, 157–189.

Locker, D. (1983) *Disability and Disadvantage*. Tavistock Publications London.

Lonsdale, S. (1990) *Women and Disability: The experiences of disability among women.* Macmillan, London.

Loucks, E.B., Berkman, L.F., Gruenewald, T.L., Seeman, T.E. (2006) Relation of social integration to inflammatory marker concentrations in men and women 70 to 79 years. *American Journal of Cardiology*, **97** (7), 1010–1016.

Lowe, B.D., Freivalds, A. (1999) The effect of carpal tunnel syndrome on group force coordination on hand tools. *Ergonomics*, **42** (4), 550–564.

Lucas, K., Lloyd, B. (2005) *Health Promotion: Evidence and experience.* Sage, London.

Lundberg, O., Nyström Peck, M. (1994) Sense of coherence, social structure and health. *European Journal of Public Health*, **4** (4), 252–257.

McAvay, G., Seeman, T., Rodin, J. (1996) A longitudinal study of change in domain specific self efficacy among older adults. *Journals of Gerontology: Series B, Psychological Sciences and Social Sciences*, **51**, 243–253.

McCrae, R.R., Costa, P.J., Jr. (1987) Validation of the five factor model of personality across instruments and observers. *Journal of Personality and Social Psychology*, **52**, 81–90.

Macdonald, E., Capewell, S. (2001) Podiatry: Cinderella speciality in search of a glass slipper? *Podiatry Now*, **4** (11), 518–520.

McEwan, B.S. (1998) Protective and damaging effects of stress mediators. *New England Journal of Medicine*, **338** (3), 171–179.

McEwan, B.S., Stellar, E. (1993) Stress and the individual mechanisms leading to disease. *Archive of Internal Medicine*, **153** (18), 2093–2101.

MacIntyre, J., Joy, E. (2000) The athletic woman: Foot and ankle injuries in dance. *Clinics in Sports Medicine*, **19** (2), 351–368.

McLoughlin, B. (1996) *Developing Psychodynamic Counselling*, (2nd edn.). Sage, London.

McReynolds, M. (1995) Rehabilitation management of the lower extremity in HIV disease. *Journal of the American Podiatric Medical Association*, **85** (7), 394–401.

Mandy, A. (2000) Burnout and work stress in newly qualified podiatrists in the NHS. *British Journal of Podiatry*, **3** (2), 31–34.

Mandy, A., McInnes, J., Bryant, E. (2007) Patterns of employment of podiatrists following graduation: A five year retrospective study. *British Journal of Podiatry*, **10** (2), 39–44.

Mandy, P. (2000) *The nature and status of chiropody and dentistry*. DPhil. thesis, Sussex University.

Mandy, P. (2008) Demons and slaves: Autonomy and status in professional practice. *Podiatry Now*, **11** (5), 23–25.

Marcantoni, C., Ortalda, V., Lupo, A., Maschio, G. (1998) Progression of renal failure in diabetic nephropathy. *Nephrology Dialysis Transplantation*, **13** (suppl. 8), 16–19.

Marcia, J. (1966) Development and validation of ego-identity status. *Journal of Personality and Social Psychology*, **3**, 551–558.

Marmot, M.G., Davey-Smith, G., Stansfield, S., Patel, C., North, F., Head, J. (1991) Health inequalities among British civil servants: The Whitehall II study. *The Lancet*, **337**, 1387–1393.

Marshall, M.A., Hamilton, W.G. (1992) Cuboid subluxations in ballet dancers. *American Journal of Sports Medicine*, **20** (2), 169–175.

Maslow, A.H. (1954) *Motivation and Personality*, (2nd edn.). Harper & Row, New York.

Maslow, A.H. (1970) *Towards a Psychology of Being*. Van Nostrand, New York.

May, C., Dowrick, C., Richardson, M. (2003) The social construction of therapeutic relationships in general medical practice. *Sociological Review*, **44** (2), 187–203.

MedicineNet.com (2009) Introduction to Dementia, http://www.medicinenet.com/dementia/article.htm, accessed 20 February 2009.

Memar, O., Cirelli, R., Lee, P., Tyring, S. (1995) Cutaneous manifestations of HIV-1 infection. *Journal of the American Podiatric Medical Association*, **85** (7), 362–373.

Mendes de Leon, C.F., Glass, T.A., Beckett, L.A., Seeman, T.E., Evans, D.A., Berkman, L.F. (1999) Social networks and disability transitions across eight intervals of yearly data in the New Haven EPESE. *Journals of Gerontology: Series B, Psychological Sciences and Social Sciences*, **54** (3), S162–S172.

Merriman, L. (1993) What is the purpose of chiropody services? *Journal of British Podiatric Medicine*, **48** (8), 121–128.

Merton, R.K., Bloom, S., Rogoff, N. (1956) Columbia/Pennsylvania studies in the sociology of medical education. *Journal of Medical Education*, **31** (8), 552–565.

Miller, S.M. (1980) When is a little information a dangerous thing? Coping with stressful events by monitoring and blunting. In: *Coping and Health*, (eds S. Levine, H. Ursin). Plenum Press, New York.

Miller, W., Rollnick, S. (2002) *Motivational Interviewing: Preparing people for change*. Guilford Press, New York.

Miller, W.R., Benefield, R.G., Tonigan, J.S. (1993) Enhancing motivation for change in problem drinking: A controlled comparison of two therapist styles. *Journal of Consulting and Clinical Psychology*, **61** (3), 455–61.

Miller, W.R., Marlatt, G.A. (1977) The Banff skiism screening test: An instrument for assessing degree of addiction. *Addictive Behaviors*, **2**, 81–82.

Miller, W.R., Rollnick, S. (1991) *Motivational Interviewing: Preparing people to change addictive behaviour*. Guilford Press, New York.

Mitchell, M. (1997) Patients' perceptions of pre-operative preparation for day surgery. *Journal of Advanced Nursing*, **26** (2), 356–363.

Mogensen, C.E. (1999) Microalbuminuria, blood pressure and diabetic renal disease: Origin and development of ideas. *Diabetologia*, **42**, 263–285.

Mokdad, A.H., Ford, E.S., Bowman, B.A. *et al.* (2000) Diabetes trends in the US: 1990–1998. *Diabetes Care*, **23**, 1278–1283.

Molitch, M.E., DeFronzo, R.A., Franz, M.J. *et al.* (2004) Nephropathy in diabetes. *Diabetes Care*, **27** (suppl. 1), S79–S83.

Moore, J., Phipps, K., Marcer, D., Lewith, G. (1985) Why do people seek treatment by alternative medicine? *British Medical Journal*, **290** (6461), 28–29.

Morgan, M. (1991) The doctor–patient relationship. In: *Sociology as Applied to Medicine*, (ed. G. Scambler). Croom Helm, Beckenham.

Morgan, M., Calnan, M., Manning, N. (1985) *Sociological Approaches to Health and Medicine*. Croom Helm, Beckenham.

Moscovici, S. (1973) Foreword. In: *Health and Illness: A social psychological analysis*, (ed. C. Herzlich). Academic Press, London.

Muggleton, J.M., Alklen, R., Chappell, P.H. (1999) Hand and arm injuries associated with repetitive manual work in industry: A review of disorders, risk factors and preventative measures. *Ergonomics*, **42** (5), 714–739.

Murphy, R.F. (1999) The damaged self. In: *Health, Illness and Healing*, (eds K. Charmaz, D.A. Paterniti). Roxbury, Los Angeles.

Murphy-Taylor, C. (1999) Children's nursing: The benefits of preparing children and parents for day surgery. *British Journal of Nursing*, **8** (12), 801–804.

Nancarrow, S.A., Borthwick, A.M. (2005) Dynamic professional boundaries in the healthcare workforce. *Sociology of Health & Illness*, **27** (7), 897–919.

Nelson, D.P. (1996) *Validity Concerns in Previous Studies Examining the Frequency of Anorexia Nervosa in Ballet Dancers*. Microform Publications International Institute for Sport and Human Performance, University of Oregon.

Nettleton, S. (2006) *Sociology of Health and Illness*. Polity Press, Cambridge.

Neuberger, G.B. (2000) The educated patient: new challenges for the medical profession. *Journal of Internal Medicine*, **247** (1), 6–10.

Neuberger, G.B., Aaronson, L.S., Gajewski, B. *et al.* (2007) Predictors of exercise and effects of exercise on symptoms, function, aerobic fitness and disease outcomes of rheumatoid arthritis. *Arthritis Care & Research*, **57** (6), 943–952.

Neugebauer, A., Katz, P.P. (2004) Impact of social support on valued activity disability and depressive symptoms in patients with rheumatoid arthritis. *Arthritis Care and Research*, **51** (4), 586–592.

Newell S.G., Woodie A. (1981) Cuboid syndrome. *Physician of Sports Medicine*, **9** (4), 71–76.

Nishizawa, K., Iijima, M., Tokita, A., Yamashiro, Y. (2001) Bone mineral density of eating disorder Nippon Rinsho. *Japanese Journal of Clinical Medicine*, **59** (3), 554–560.

Noyes, R., Jr., Hartz, A.J., Doebbeling, C.C. *et al.* (2000) Illness fears in the general population. *Psychosomatic Medicine*, **62** (3), 318–325.

Osterman, K., Kottkamp, R. (1993) *Reflective Practice for Educators: Improving schooling through professional development*. Corwin Press, Newbury Park, CA.

Palmer, M. (1997) *Freud and Jung on Religion*. Routledge, London and New York.

Pargament, K.I., Koenig, H.G., Tarakeshwar, N., Hahn, J. (2001) Religious struggle as a predictor of mortality among medically ill elderly patients: A two year longitudinal study. *Archives of Internal Medicine*, **161** (15), 1881–1885.

Parkes, C.M. (1986) *Bereavement: Studies in grief in adult life*, (3rd edn.). Tavistock, London.

Parsons, T. (1939) *The Professions and Social Structure in Essays in Sociological Theory*. Free Press, New York.

Parsons, T. (1951) *The Social System*. The Free Press, Glencoe, IL.

Parving, H.H., Osterby, R., Ritz, E. (2000) Diabetic nephropathy. In: *The Kidney*, (ed. B.M. Brenner). W.B. Saunders, Philadelphia.

Paterson, C., Britten, N. (1999) 'Doctors can't help much': The search for an alternative. *British Journal of General Practice*, **49** (445), 626–629.

Paton, D., Brown, R. (1991) *Lifespan Health Psychology: Nursing: Problems and interventions*. Harper Collins, London.

Pearson, M., Michell, L. (2000) Smoke rings: Social network analysis of friendship groups, smoking and drug-taking. *Drugs Education, Prevention and Policy*, **7** (1), 21–37.

Pennebaker, J. (1982) *The Psychology of Physical Symptoms*. Springer Verlag, New York.

Peralta, V., Cuesta, M.J., de Leon, J. (1991) Premorbid personality and positive and negative symptoms in schizophrenia. *Acta Psychiatrica Scandinavica*, **84** (4), 336–339.

Peterson, A. (2001) *A Will to Win*. Macmillan, London.

Pew-Fetzer (1994) *Health Professions Education and Relationship-Centered Care: Report of the Pew-Fetzer Task Force on Advancing Psychosocial Health Education*. Pew Health Professions Commission, San Francisco.

Pheasant, S. (1994) *Ergonomics, Work and Health*. Macmillan, London.

Phillimore, P., Beattie, A.P. (1994) The widening gap: Inequality of health in northern England 1981–1991. *British Medical Journal*, **308** (6937), 1125–1128.

Phillips, C. (1999) Strength training of dancers during the adolescent growth spurt. *Journal of Dance Medicine and Science*, **3**, 66–72.

Pierce, J.P., Farkas, A., Zhu, S.H., Berry, C., Kaplan, R.M. (1996) Should the stage of change model be challenged? *Addiction*, **91**, 1290–1292.

Pietroni, P.C. (1991) Stereotypes or archetypes? A study of perceptions amongst health-care students. *Journal of Social Work Practice*, **5** (1), 61–69.

Piggott, A.E. (1991) A study into the incidence and prevalence of self reported back pain amongst chiropody students and 1986 graduates. *Journal of British Podiatric Medicine*, **46**, 83–87.

Pitts, M. (1991) The experience of treatment. In: *The Psychology of Health*, (eds M. Pitts, K. Phillips). Routledge, London.

Povey, R., Conner, M., Sparks, P., James, R., Sheppard, R. (2000) Application of the theory of planned behaviour to two dietary behaviours: Roles of perceived control and self efficacy. *British Journal of Health Psychology*, **5**, 121–139.

Powers, A. (2001) Diabetes mellitus. In: *Harrison's Principles of Internal Medicine*, (eds E. Braunwald, A.S. Fauci, D.L. Kasper) *et al.* McGraw-Hill, New York.

Prigerson, H.G., Bierhals, A.J., Kasel, S.V. *et al.* (1997) Traumatic grief as a risk factor for mental and physical morbidity. *American Journal of Psychiatry*, **154** (5), 616–623.

Prochaska, J.O., DiClemente, C.C. (1983) Transtheoretical therapy: Toward a more integrative model of change. *Psychotherapy Theory Research and Practice*, **19** (3), 276–288.

Quill, T.E., Brody, H. (1996) Physician recommendations and patient autonomy: Finding a balance between physician power and patient choice. *Annals of Internal Medicine*, **125** (9), 763–769.

Qureshi, H., Walker, A. (1989) *The Caring Relationship: Elderly people and their families*. Macmillan, London.

Ramsay, R., de Groot, W. (1977) A further look at bereavement. Paper presented at EATI Conference, Uppsala, (cited in Hodgkinson, P.E. (1980) Treating abnormal grief in the bereaved. *Nursing Times*, **17 January**, 126–128).

Randall, G., Brown, S. (1994) *Falling Out: A research study of homeless ex-service people*. Crisis, London.

Reynolds-Whyte, S., Ingstad, B. (1995) Disability and culture: An overview. In: *Disability and Culture*, (eds S. Reynolds-Whyte, B. Ingstad). University of California Press.

Roberts, A.H., Kewman, D.G., Mercier, L., Hovell, M. (1993) The power of nonspecific effects in healing: Implications for psychosocial and biological treatments. *Clinical Psychology Review*, **13**, 375–391.

Roberts, R., Towell, T., Golding, J. (2001) *Foundations of Health Psychology*. Palgrave, Basingstoke.

Rocchiccioli, J.T., O'Donoghue, C.R., Buttigieg, S. (2005) Diabetes in Malta: Current findings and future trends. *Malta Medical Journal*, **17** (1), 16–19.

Roderick, P.J., Raleigh, V.S., Hallam, L., Mallick, N.P. (1996) The need and demand for renal replacement therapy in ethnic minorities in England. *Journal of Epidemiology and Community Health*, **50** (3), 334–339.

Rogers, C. (1951) *Client-Centered Therapy*. Houghton Mifflin, Boston.

Rogers, W.A. (2002) *Evidence-based Medicine in Practice: Limiting or facilitating patient choice?* Blackwell, Oxford.

Rotter, J.B. (1966) Generalised expectancies for the internal versus external control of reinforcement theory. *Psychological Monographs*, **901**, 1–28.

Russell, G. (1999) *Essential Psychology*. Routledge, London.

Russell, S. (1996) Ability to pay for health care concepts and evidence. *Health Policy Plan*, **11** (3), 219–237.

Ryan, R.M., Deci, E.L., Grolnick, W.S. (1995) Autonomy, relatedness and the self: Their relation to development and psychopathology. In: *Developmental Psychopathology*, (eds D. Cicchetti, D.J. Cohen). John Wiley & Sons, New York.

Sapolsky, R.M. (1996) Why stress is bad for your brain. *Science*, **273** (5276), 749–750.

Sasco, A.J., Kleihues, P. (1999) Why can't we convince the young not to smoke? *European Journal of Cancer*, **35** (14), 1933–1940.

Sauter, S., Hurrell, J., Jr., Cooper, C. (1989) *Job Control and Worker Health*. John Wiley & Sons, New York.

Savona-Ventura, C. (2005) *Contemporary Medicine in Malta (1798–1979)*. Publishers Enterprises Group (PEG), Malta.

Schaefer, C., Coyne, J.C., Lazarus, R.S. (1981) The health related functions of social support. *Journal of Behavioral Medicine*, **4**, 381–406.

Scharloo, M., Kapstein, A.A., Weinman, J. *et al.* (1998) Illness perceptions, coping and functioning in patients with rheumatoid arthritis, chronic obstructive pulmonary disease and psoriasis. *Journal of Psychosomatic Medicine*, **44**, 573–585.

Schartzbaum, A., McGrath, J., Rothman, R. (1973) The perception of prestige differences amongst medical specialities. *Social Science and Medicine*, **7**, 365–371.

Schneiderman, L.J., Jecker, N.S., Jonsen, A.R. (1990) Medical futility: Its meaning and ethical implications. *Annals of Internal Medicine*, **112**, 949–951.

Seeman, P., Lee, T., Chau-Wong, M., Wong, K. (1976) Antipsychotic drug doses and neuroleptic/dopamine receptors. *Nature*, **261**, 717–719.

Seeman, T.E., Kaplan, G.A., Knudsen, L., Cohen, R., Guralnik, J. (1987) Social network ties and mortality among the elderly in the Alameda County study. *American Journal of Epidemiology*, **126** (4), 714–723.

Senge, P.M. (1990) *The Fifth Discipline: The art and practice of the learning organization.* Doubleday, New York.

Senior, M., Viveash, B. (1998) *Health and Illness.* Macmillan, London.

Seyle, H. (1950) *The Physiology and Pathology of Exposure to Stress,* Acta, Montreal.

Shaw, C.J., Shaw, T.F., Bowden, P. (2001) Study to determine the incidence of musculoskeletal complaints amongst podiatry students at Salford University. *British Journal of Podiatry*, **4** (4), 120–123.

Silverman, P.R., Worden, J.W. (1993) Children's reactions to death of a parent. In: *Handbook of Bereavement: Theory, research and intervention*, (eds M.S. Stroebe, V. Stroebe, R.O. Hansson). Cambridge University Press, New York.

Simmons, R.G., Blyth, D.A., McKinney, K.L. (1983) The social and psychological effects of puberty on white females. In: *Girls and Puberty: Biological and psychological perspectives*, (eds J. Brooks-Gunn, A.C. Petersen). Plenum Press, New York.

Singh, N., Armstrong, D.G., Lipsky, B.A. (2005) Preventing foot ulcers in patients with diabetes. *Journal of the American Medical Association*, **293** (2), 217–228.

Siris, S.G. (2001) Suicide and schizophrenia. *Journal of Psychopharmacology*, **15** (2), 127–135.

Smith, K., Skelton, H., Yeager, J. *et al.* (1994) Cutaneous findings in HIV-1 positive patients: A 42 month prospective study. *Journal of the American Academy of Dermatology*, **31** (5), 746–754.

Soltani, S., Kenyon, E., Barbosa, P. (1996) Chronic and aggressive plantar verrucae in a patient with HIV. *Journal of the American Podiatric Medical Association*, **86** (11) 555–558.

Spiegel, D. (1991) Second thoughts on personality, stress, and disease. *Psychological Inquiry*, **2** (3), 266–268.

Stamler, J., Vaccaro, O., Neaton, J.D., Wentworth, D. (1993) Diabetes: Other risk factors and 12 year cardiovascular mortality for men screened in the Multiple Risk Factor Intervention Trial. *Diabetes Care*, **16**, 434–444.

Stepney, R. (1981) Habits and addictions. *Bulletin of the British Psychological Society*, **34**, 233–235.

Steptoe, A. (1997) Stress management. In: *Cambridge Handbook of Psychology, Health and Medicine*, (eds A. Baum, S. Newman, J. Weinman, R. West, C. McManus). Cambridge University Press.

Stockwell, T. (1996) Interventions cannot ignore intentions. *Addiction*, **91**, 1283–1284.

Storch, J., Stinson, S. (1988) Concepts of deprofessionalisation with application to nursing. In: *Politics in Nursing: Past, present and future: Volume 3*, (ed. R. White). John Wiley & Sons, Chichester.

Stroebe, M.S. (2001) Bereavement research and theory: Retrospective and prospective. *American Behavioral Scientist*, **44** (5), 854–865.

Stroebe, M.S., Stroebe, W., Hansson, R.O. (1993) Contemporary themes and controversies in bereavement research. In: *Handbook of Bereavement: Theory, research and intervention*, (eds M.S. Stroebe, W. Stroebe, R.O. Hansson). Cambridge University Press, New York.

Susman, J. (1994) Disability: stigma and deviance. *Social Science and Medicine*, **38** (1), 15–22.

Sutton, R., Kahn, R.L. (1984) Prediction, understanding, and control as antidotes to organizational stress. In: *Handbook of Organizational Behavior*, (ed. J. Lorsch). Harvard University Press.

Sutton, S. (1998) How ordinary people in Great Britain perceive the health risks of smoking. *Journal of Epidemiology and Community Health*, **52** (5), 338–339.

Sutton, S.R. (1996) Further support for the stages of change model? *Addiction*, **91**, 1287–1289.

Szasz, T.S., Hollender, M.S. (1956) A contribution to the philosophy of medicine. *Archives of Internal Medicine*, **97**, 585–592.

Taylor, S.E. (1986) *Health Psychology*. Random House, New York.

Terry. D.J., O'Leary, J.E. (1995) The theory of planned behaviour: The effects of perceived behavioural control and self efficacy. *British Journal of Social Psychology*, **34** (2), 199–220.

Thoits, P.A. (1994) The sociology of emotions. *Annual Reviews of Sociology*, **15**, 317–342.

Thomas, K., Carr, J., Westlake, L., Williams, B. (1991) Use of non-orthodox and conventional healthcare in Great Britain. *British Medical Journal*, **302** (6770), 207–210.

Townsend, P. (1962) *The Last Refuge: A survey of residential institutions and homes for the aged in England and Wales*. Routledge & Kegan Paul, London.

Townsend, P., Davidson, N. (eds). (1982) *Inequalities in Health: The Black Report*. Penguin Books, Harmondsworth.

Treaster, D.E., Burr, D. (2004) Gender differences in prevalence of upper extremity musculoskeletal disorders. *Ergonomics*, **47** (5), 495–525.

US Renal Data System (2000) *Annual Data Report*. National Institutes of Health, National Institute of Diabetes and Digestive and Kidney Diseases, Minneapolis..

Vincent, C., Furnham, A. (1997) The perceived efficacy of complementary and orthodox medicine: A replication. *Complementary Therapies in Medicine*, **5**, 85–89.

Vora, A.R., Yeoman, C.M., Hayter, J.P. (2000) Oral cancer: Alcohol tobacco and paan use and understanding of oral cancer risk among Asian males in Leicester. *British Dental Journal*, **188**, 441–451.

Walker, E.A., Katon, W.J. (1990) Psychological stress affecting physical conditions and responses to stress. In: *Clinical Psychiatry for Medical Students*, (ed. A. Stoudemire). J.B. Lippincott, Philadelphia.

Wallstone, K.A. Wallstone, B.S. (1978) Development of the multidimensional health locus of control (MHLC). *Health Education Monographs*, **6**, 160–170.

Waterman, A.S. (1982) Identity development from adolescent to adulthood: An extension of theory and a review of research. *Developmental Psychology*, **18**, 341–348.

Weiner, B. (1986) *An Attribution Theory of Motivation and Emotion*. Springer Verlag, New York.

Wenger, G.C., Shahtahmasebi, S. (1990) Variations in support networks: Some policy implications. In: *Aiding and Ageing: The coming crisis*, (ed. J. Mogey). Greenwood Press, Westport, CT.

Wenger, W.C. (1994) Support networks and dementia. *International Journal of Geriatric Psychiatry*, **9**, 181–194.

Weston, D. (1996) *Psychology: Mind, Brain and Culture*. John Wiley & Sons, New York.

Wilensky, H.L. (1964) The professionalisation of everyone. *American Journal of Sociology*, **70** (2), 137–158.

Wiles, R., Higgins, J. (1996) Doctor–patient relationships in the private sector: Patients' perceptions. *Sociology of Health and Illness*, **18** (3), 341–356.

Wilkinson, R.G. (1997) *Unhealthy Societies: The afflictions of inequality*. Routledge, London.

Williams, G.C., Grow, V.M., Freedman, Z., Ryan, R.M., Deci, E.L. (1996) Motivational predictors of weight loss and weight-loss maintenance. *Journal of Personality & Social Psychology*, **70**, 115–26.

Worden, J.W. (1991) *Grief Counseling and Grief Therapy: Handbook for the mental health practitioner*, (2nd edn.). Springer, New York.

World Health Organization (1980) *The International Classification of Impairments, Disabilities, and Handicaps*. WHO, Geneva.

World Health Organization (1999) *Definition, Diagnosis and Classification of Diabetes Mellitus and its Complications*. WHO Consultation, Geneva.

Young, A., Dinan, S. (2005) Activity in later life. *British Medical Journal* **330** (7484), 189–191.

Zborowski, M. (1952) Cultural components in response to pain. *Journal of Social Issues*, **8** (4), 16–30.

Ziebland, S., Fitzpatrick, R., Jenkinson, C. (1993) Tacit models of disability underlying health status instruments. *Social Science and Medicine*, **37** (1), 69–75.

Index